Christer Ahlström

Phonocardiographic Signal Processing

Christer Ahlström

Phonocardiographic Signal Processing

A Nonlinear Approach

VDM Verlag Dr. Müller

Impressum

Bibliografische Information der Deutschen Nationalbibliothek: Die Deutsche Nationalbibliothek verzeichnet diese Publikation in der Deutschen Nationalbibliografie; detaillierte bibliografische Daten sind im Internet über http://dnb.d-nb.de abrufbar.

Coverbild: www.purestockx.com

Erscheinungsjahr: 2008
Erscheinungsort: Saarbrücken

Verlag:
VDM Verlag Dr. Müller Aktiengesellschaft & Co. KG, Dudweiler Landstr. 125 a, 66123 Saarbrücken, Deutschland,
Telefon +49 681 9100-698, Telefax +49 681 9100-988,
Email: info@vdm-verlag.de
Zugl.: Linköping, Linköping University, Dept. of Biomedical Engineering, PhD dissertation, 2008

Herstellung:
Schaltungsdienst Lange o.H.G., Zehrensdorfer Str. 11, D-12277 Berlin
Books on Demand GmbH, Gutenbergring 53, D-22848 Norderstedt

ISBN: 978-3-639-07110-8

To my lovely sunshine Anneli.

*You are all I want and everything I need.
Thank you for keeping me happy.*

Table of Contents

Preface

Using sounds from the body to assess the health status of a patient is one of the oldest diagnostic techniques. The history of auscultation, or listening to the sounds of the body, can be described as a few evolutionary leaps. Hippocrates (460–377 BC) provided the foundation for auscultation by simply putting his ear against the chest of a patient. The next leap was made by Robert Hooke (1635–1703) who realized the diagnostic potential of cardiac auscultation. The biggest breakthrough came in 1816 when René Laennec (1781–1826) invented the stethoscope, the most widely spread diagnostic instrument in the history of biomedical engineering.

New advances in cardiac imaging, such as echocardiography and magnetic resonance imaging, have become so dominating in cardiac assessment that the main use of cardiac auscultation is nowadays as a preliminary test in the primary health care. These more recent techniques provide more accurate results, but they also require expensive equipment and skilled personnel. In a world where modern health care is striving for cost contained point-of-care testing, it is now time to bring cardiac auscultation up to date. Decision support systems based on heart sounds and murmurs would improve the accuracy of auscultation by providing objective additional information, and the overall aim of this book is to present signal processing tools able to extract such information. This book will not delve deeply into certain important areas in phonocardiographic (PCG) signal processing such as classification, artificial neural networks and evolutionary computing. Instead, the main foci will be on feature extraction and feature selection, especially by using recent nonlinear techniques.

This book is a slightly modified version of my PhD thesis [6]. The thesis, and consequently also the book, is thus profoundly influenced by my own research. In fact, five research papers provide the backbone of the book. Unfortunately, these papers were not entirely (chrono)logically ordered. For example, studies on aortic stenosis (AS) [8] and mitral insufficiency (MI) [141] should have preceded the study where these two cardiac defects were distinguished from each other [11]. This is however not the case. This transposed time line resulted in the fact that the auto mutual information (AMI) feature was not part of the AS assessment study and that AMI, sample entropy and the correlation dimension were "left out" from paper [11]. Clearly, it would have been very interesting to include all of the features in paper [11], but I simply did not know of these techniques back then. This is also the reason why the study underlying paper [11] precedes both paper [8] and paper [141] and why human experiments were conducted before studies on dogs were performed. Despite this dilemma, I hope you will enjoy reading the book. It contains a whole lot of interesting information about phonocardiographic signal processing.

v

Contents overview
Chapters 1–3 provides introductory information about anatomy, physiology, PCG signals and signal processing theory. The emphasis in chapter 3 is on signal analysis and especially on the task of extracting descriptive features. Related issues such as noise reduction, classification, feature selection and system evaluation are also mentioned. This chapter is written in a general manner free from cardiac sound examples, so if the reader is familiar with the material it is possible to skip it altogether. Chapter 4 describes direct and indirect heart sound localization and briefly mentions heart sound segmentation. A rigorous survey of available indirect heart sound localization methods is given and a comparative performance evaluation is presented. A section on S3 detection is also included. Segmentation of PCG signals into S1, systole, S2 and diastole is an important preprocessing step in most PCG signal processing applications. Chapter 5 describes murmur classification and assessment, starting with AS and MI, and concluding with classification of MI, AS and physiological murmurs. Chapter 6 makes use of methodology introduced in chapter 4 to find and remove heart sounds to make lung sounds more audible. More specifically, recurrence time statistics and nonlinear prediction are used for the actual heart sound cancellation process. Chapter 7 also makes use of methodology from chapter 4 to derive cardiac time intervals. The time intervals reflect certain processes in the cardiovascular system and facilitate indirect tracking of blood pressure changes and monitoring of respiration in a noninvasive, non-obstructive and non-intrusive manner. Chapter 8 contains a discussion about PCG signal processing in general, particularly regarding future aspects.

Acknowledgements

Interdisciplinary research requires expertise from many different fields of knowledge, and I am very fortunate to have colleagues and friends who have helped me in the writing of this book.

This work would not have been possible without my former supervisors. Per Ask (Linköping) is a pioneer in biomedical engineering and his experience has been priceless. Thank you for having faith in my ideas and for allowing me to go where it was sometimes hard to follow. Anders Johansson (Linköping) is a very professional researcher and also an excellent friend. Thank you for being my guiding light and for keeping my hopes up. Peter Hult (Linköping) introduced me to the intelligent stethoscope and the world of bioacoustics, and without his preceding work [107] I would never have had the opportunity to delve into this interesting research area.

To all of my co-workers: I would have been lost without your knowledge. Many thanks to Eva Nylander (Linköping), Linda Rattfält (Linköping), Jan-Erik Karlsson (Jönköping), Peter Rask (Örebro), Jens Häggström (Uppsala), Ulf Dahlström (Linköping), Clarence Kvart (Uppsala) and Toste Länne (Linköping) for lending me your expertise. I am particularly grateful to Katja Höglund (Uppsala) and Ingrid Ljungvall (Uppsala) for giving me the opportunity to experience a double cultural clash and to Fredrik Hasfjord (Linköping) and Olle Liljefelt (Linköping) for stimulating discussions on fractal dimensions and nonlinear gap-filling. Also many thanks to January Gnitecki (Manitoba) for giving me a badly needed exhortation which brought me back on the upright track.

I am very grateful to the kind and forthcoming personnel at the Dept. of Internal Medicine (Ryhov County Hospital), at the Dept. of Clinical Physiology (Örebro University Hospital) and at the Dept. of Clinical Physiology (Linköping University Hospital), for all help and persistent support regarding data acquisition. I am also very grateful to the Uppsala research group at the Swedish University of Agricultural Sciences for letting me use their database of PCG signals from dogs.

Many thanks to Leif Sörnmo (Lund) who acted as an opponent during my Licentiate degree examination [5] and who tutored me while I was reading his excellent book [217]. Also many thanks to Pablo Laguna (Zaragoza) who was my opponent during my PhD dissertation and hence made sure that many or the typos and errors in my thesis [6] did not make it into this book.

Finally, I am very fortunate to have the best of friends. Linda for sharing her boggling and sometimes windswept thoughts, Jonas for keeping me down to earth and Markus for keeping up with my complaints. I also owe a great deal to Amir, my office mate whom I trust with my life. Finally, my sincerest gratitude goes to my family for all their support over the years.

This work was supported by grants from the Swedish Agency for Innovation Systems, the Health Research Council in the South-East of Sweden, the Swedish Research Council, the Swedish Heart-Lung Foundation and the NIMED Center of Excellence.

Christer Ahlström
Linköping, 2008

Abbreviations

AMI	Auto mutual information
AR	Auto regressive
ARMA	Auto regressive moving average
AS	Aortic valve stenosis
AV	Atrioventricular
CCI	Cross correlation index
COPD	Chronic obstructive pulmonary disease
D_2	Correlation dimension
ECG	Electrocardiographic signal
EMAT	Electromechanical activation time
LBNP	Lower body negative pressure
MA	Moving average
MI	Mitral insufficiency (mitral regurgitation)
MRI	Magnetic resonance imaging
PCG	Phonocardiographic signal
PEP	Pre-ejection period
PPG	Photoplethysmographic signal
PSD	Power spectral density
S1	The first heart sound
S2	The second heart sound
S3	The third heart sound
S4	The fourth heart sound
SBP	Systolic blood pressure
SFFS	Sequential floating forward selection
SVD	Singular Value Decomposition
T1	Recurrence time of the first kind
T2	Recurrence time of the second kind
VFD	Variance fractal dimension

1

Introduction

"When an examination is an art, decisions about health, disease,
and its treatment can only be arbitrary or subjective."
Howard H. Wayne

The stethoscope is a recognized icon for the medical profession, and for a long time, physicians have relied on auscultation for detection and characterization of cardiac disease. New advances in cardiac imaging have however changed this picture. Echocardiography and magnetic resonance imaging (MRI) have become so dominating in cardiac assessment that the main use of cardiac auscultation is nowadays as a preliminary test in the primary health care. Basically, all patients presenting anything but normal auscultatory findings are sent to a cardiology clinic for further investigations. In a world where modern health care is striving for cost contained point-of-care testing, it is now time to bring cardiac auscultation up to date. Decision support systems based on heart sounds and murmurs would improve the accuracy of auscultation by providing objective additional information, and the overall aim of this book is to present signal processing tools able to extract such information.

This introductory chapter will provide a peak preview of upcoming chapters. Heart sounds and murmurs will be introduced and a number of phonocardiographic (PCG) signal processing examples will be given. Terminology and methodology will be used rather carelessly in this chapter, but every example contains pointers to other chapters where more information is available.

There are six data sets which this book relies upon. Some of these data sets are used more than once why they will all be surveyed in this chapter.

1.1 Preliminaries on cardiac sounds

Aristotle found the heart to be the seat of intelligence, motion and sensation. Other organs surrounding the heart, such as the brain and the lungs, merely existed as cooling devices [66]. Since the fourth century BC, our understanding of the heart has changed its role from an all-embracing organ towards a highly specialized device

1

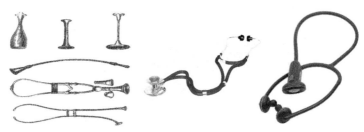

Fig. 1.1: **Early monaural stethoscopes (top left), Cummann's and Allison's stetho-scopes (lower left), a modern binaural stethoscope (middle) and a modern electronic stethoscope, Meditron M30 (right).**

whose purpose is to propel blood. Knowledge about auscultation has evolved along-side with discoveries about heart function. Robert Hooke (1635–1703), an English polymath, was the first to realize the diagnostic potential of cardiac auscultation:

> *I have been able to hear very plainly the beating of a man's heart ... Who knows, I say, but that it may be possible to discover the motion of the internal parts of bodies ... by the sound they make; one may discover the works performed in several offices and shops of a man's body and thereby discover what instrument is out of order.*

When René Laennec (1781–1826) invented the stethoscope in 1816, cardiac aus-cultation became a fundamental clinical tool and remains so today. A selection of stethoscopes from different eras is presented in figure 1.1.

Normally there are two heart sounds, S1 and S2, produced concurrently with the closure of the atrioventricular valves and the semilunar valves, respectively. A third and a fourth heart sound, S3 and S4, might also exist. Additionally, a variety of other sounds such as heart murmurs or adventitious sounds may be present. Heart murmurs can be innocent or pathologic, and they are especially common among children (50-80% of the population has murmurs during childhood, but only about 1% of these murmurs are pathological [181]) and in the elderly (prevalence estimates range from 29%–60% [48, 212]). Most common are murmurs originating from the left side of the heart, especially aortic valve stenosis (AS) and mitral insufficiency (MI). A more thorough review of the origin of heart sounds and murmurs can be found in chapter 2.

It is often during auscultation that murmurs are detected. Performing auscultation is however difficult since it is based on the physician's ability to perceive and interpret a variety of low-intensity and low-frequency sounds, see figure 1.2. Auscultation is also highly subjective and even the nomenclature used to describe the sounds varies amongst clinicians. Unfortunately, the auscultatory skills amongst physicians demonstrate a negative trend. The loss has occurred despite new teaching aids such as multimedia tutorials, and the main reasons are the availability of new diagnostic tools such as echocardiography and MRI, a lack of confidence and increased concern about litigations [181]. An automatic decision support system able to screen and assess the PCG signal would thus be both time and cost saving while relieving many patients from needless anxiety.

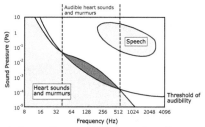

Fig. 1.2: Relationship between the acoustic range of cardiac sounds and the threshold of audibility of the human ear. Figure redrawn from Leatham [132].

1.2 Preliminaries on PCG signal processing

The PCG signal discloses information about cardiac function through vibrations caused by the working heart. In the early days of PCG signal analysis, manual interpretation of waveform patterns was performed in the time domain. Heart sounds were identified as composite oscillations related to valve closure and heart murmurs seemed to derive from malfunctioning valves or from abnormal holes in the septal wall. When the Fourier transform became practically useful, it provided further information about periodicity and the distribution of signal power. In many biomedical signals, the Fourier transform showed that sharp frequency peaks were rare, and when they did exist, they often indicated disease [79]. The PCG signal turned out to be different. Murmurs possessed characteristics similar to colored noise, and with increasing disease severity, the frequency spectrum became more and more complicated. In an attempt to disentangle the frequency spectrum, joint time-frequency analysis was employed [155]. In later studies, it could be shown that heart sounds consisted of several components where each component had a main frequency that varied with time. This short introduction basically brings us up to date regarding the tools used for PCG signal analysis. In this book, nonlinear techniques will be investigated as means to explore the PCG signal even further.

Heart sounds and murmurs are of relatively low intensity and are band-limited to about 10–1000 Hz, see figure 1.2. Meanwhile the human auditory system, which is adapted to speech, is unable to take in much of this information. An automated signal processing system, equipped with a sound sensor, would be able to exploit this additional information. In a clinical setting, the main tasks for such a system would be to:

- Emphasize the audibility of the PCG signal.
- Extract or emphasize weak or abnormal events in the PCG signal.
- Extract information suitable for assessment and classification of heart diseases.

Emphasize the audibility of the PCG signal
Noise is a big problem in PCG recordings. The sensor, the sensor contact surface, the patient's position, the auscultation area, the respiration phase and the background noise all influence the quality of the sound. In practice this means that the recordings often contain noise such as friction rubs, rumbling sounds from the stomach, respiratory sounds from the lungs and background noise from the clinical environment. Most of these noise sources have their frequency content in the same range as the signal of interest, why linear filters are not very suitable. In figure 1.3a, a very noisy PCG signal is shown. Wavelet denoising, which will be introduced in section 3.7 and used on PCG signals in chapter 4, somewhat emphasizes the heart sounds (figure 1.3b), but the signal is still covered in noise. When trying to emphasize S1 alone, a matched filter can be employed to improve the results, see figure 1.3c. A problem with this approach is that even though S1 occurrences are emphasized, the actual appearance of S1 is lost. Matched filtering relies on finding a representative template of, in this case, S1. Since S1 is basically triggered by the R-peak in an electrocardiogram (ECG), event related processing techniques (section 3.7) can be used to obtain this template. In chapter 4, very accurate localization of S1 is achieved by using this technique.

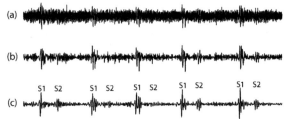

Fig. 1.3: **Example of a very noisy PCG signal (a) and the result of wavelet denoising (b). In (c), occurrences of S1 are emphasized by employing a matched filter.**

A particular noise cancellation problem is transient noise removal. Potential use in a PCG setting is to remove disturbances such as friction rubs. A related problem, where the heart sounds themselves are considered as noise, is the task of removing heart sounds with the aim to make lung sounds more audible (lung sounds is often the first resource for detection and discrimination of respiratory diseases, see chapter 6). Again, the frequency content of the noise (heart sounds) and the signal (lung sounds) are heavily overlapping. Instead of trying to filter out the heart sounds, it is possible to locate the heart sounds (chapter 4), remove them altogether and fill in the missing gaps based on time series forecasting (section 3.8). An example of a lung sound signal before and after heart sound cancellation (section 6) is given in figure 1.4.

Extract or emphasize weak or abnormal events in the PCG signal
A typical example of finding specific components in the PCG signal is the task of automatically locating S3 (section 4.5). Since S3 is of low amplitude, short duration and low frequency, it is sometimes difficult to detect during auscultation. One automatic method for extracting S3 is to look for changes in a so called recurrence

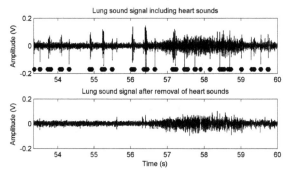

Fig. 1.4: Example of a lung sound signal before and after heart sound cancellation. The results from a heart sound localization algorithm are indicated by the bars. In this case, the patient has a third heart sound and there are also some false positive detections. In the lower plot, an error caused by the prediction algorithm can be found just before 58 seconds.

time statistic (section 3.6.2). This statistic is sensitive to changes in a reconstructed state space (section 3.4), and is particularly good at detecting weak signal transitions such as S3. An example is given in figure 1.5.

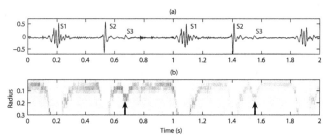

Fig. 1.5: Example of a PCG signal from a patient with a third heart sound (a). An image showing a recurrence time statistic as a function of time and a neighborhood radius clearly indicates instances of S3 (arrows in subplot b).

Extract information suitable for assessment and classification of heart diseases

The third item in the list is about finding signal representations that facilitate separation or grouping of data. Figure 1.6 shows a feature space spanned by two parameters, the correlation dimension (section 3.4.1) of a systolic murmur and the duration that the murmur has a frequency content exceeding 200 Hz. Clearly, these two parameters are almost capable of separating PCG signals containing innocent murmurs from murmurs caused by AS. The line trying to separate the groups was derived with a linear classification technique called linear discriminant analysis (section 3.9). This example shows an application with emphasis on AS classification (section 5.1). Also included in this book are methods for MI classification (section 5.2) and for classifying murmurs from different valvular diseases (section 5.3).

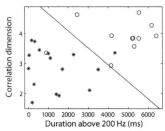

Fig. 1.6: Example of a feature space spanned by the two parameters correlation dimension and duration above 200 Hz. The circles represent murmurs caused by aortic stenosis while the stars represent innocent murmurs. The line trying to separate the two groups was derived with linear discriminant analysis.

1.3 Data sets

A number of data sets have been used in this book. The data sets, summarized in table 1.1, will be referred to by their roman numerals as data set I–VI. Since the aims of this book are focused on developing PCG signal processing techniques, full clinical trials were neither intended nor carried out. Nevertheless, to emulate the clinical situation where the system most likely will be used, the majority of the data sets were recorded in a clinical environment.

Data set I
Contains ECG, PCG and photoplethysmography (PPG) signals from ten healthy subjects (8 male, 2 female, mean age 28 years). Two measurements were however aborted because of difficulties for the subjects to adapt to the measurement situation. Data from these two subjects were excluded from the data set. The purpose of recording this data set was to investigate the correlation between certain cardiac time intervals and blood pressure as well as respiration rate, why also blood pressure and respiration were measured. The acquisition protocol consisted of five phases; a five minute resting phase, about five minutes of hypotension, five minutes of rest, about two minutes of hypertension and finally another five minutes of rest. Lower body negative pressure (LBNP) was applied to invoke hypotension [173] and isometric muscle contraction to invoke hypertension [69]. The test subjects were instructed to relax and breathe naturally throughout all measurement phases.

The ECG (Diascope DS 521, S&W Medicoteknik AS, Albertslund, Denmark, standard 3-lead placement), the PCG (Siemens E285E microphone amplifier with a Siemens EMT25C microphone, Solna, Sweden, located at the second intercostal space along the right sternal border), the PPG (Nellcor Puritan Bennett, NPB-295, Albertslud, Denmark) and the respiration reference (Optovent system, Accelerator AB, Linkoping, Sweden) were recorded and digitized with a DAQ-Card 700 from National Instruments (Austin, TX, USA, fs = 2 kHz). Blood pressure was measured with either an automatic oscillometric instrument (Datascope Accutor Plus, Paramus, NJ, USA, located on the upper left arm, n = 8) or a cannula (Becton Dickinson, Franklin Lakes, NJ, USA) positioned in the left radial artery connected

Table 1.1: **Summary of the data sets** (PCG–phonocardiography, ECG–electrocardiography, PPG–photoplethysmography).

Set	Subjects	Measured signals	f_s	Sensor	Description
I	10	ECG PCG PPG Blood pressure Respiration	2 kHz	EMT25C	10 healthy subjects (8 male, 2 female, mean age 28 years). About 20 minutes of data (5 minutes rest, about 5 minutes hypotension, 5 minutes rest, about 2 minutes hypertension and 5 minutes rest). Reference methods: Respiration monitored with Optovent, blood pressure monitored via an automatic oscillometric instrument or continuously via intraarterial cannula.
II	27	ECG PCG Echocardiography	44.1 kHz	Meditron	27 boxer dogs with various degrees of aortic stenosis (12 male, 15 female, mean age 2.15 years). 10 seconds of data recorded in a quiet room. Reference method: Aortic flow velocity via echocardiography.
III	77	ECG PCG Echocardiography	44.1 kHz	Meditron	77 small to medium-sized dogs with various degrees of mitral insufficiency (36 male, 41 female, mean age 9 years). 10 seconds of data recorded in a quiet room. Reference methods: Auscultation and echocardiography.
IV	36	ECG PCG Echocardiography	44.1 kHz	Meditron	36 patients with physiological murmurs ($n = 7$) and various degrees of aortic stenosis ($n = 23$) and mitral insufficiency ($n = 6$) (19 male, 17 female, mean age 69 years, all with native heart valves). Reference method: Echocardiography evaluated by expert.
V	6	ECG PCG	6 kHz	EMT25C	6 healthy subjects (6 male, mean age 28 years). Nearly 2 minutes of data recorded (30 s of tidal breathing, about 60 s of breathing with continuously increasing breath volumes and 10 s of breath hold). Reference method: Auscultation by expert.
VI	10	ECG PCG	2.5 kHz	EMT25C	10 healthy children (5 male, 5 female, mean age 10.5 years). 30 seconds of data recorded in a sound proof room. Reference method: PCG evaluated by expert.

to a blood pressure transducer (Abbott Critical Care Systems, Chicago, IL, USA) and connected to a monitor (Medimatic, Genoa, Italy, n = 2). The measurement setup is illustrated in figure 1.7.

All subjects were normotensive with (mean ± SD) systolic blood pressure 119 ± 8 mmHg and diastolic blood pressure 71 ± 9 mmHg ($n = 8$). LBNP reduced upper body systolic blood pressure by 24 ± 14 mmHg and the static muscle contraction increased it by 18 ± 12 mmHg.

Limitations: Intra-arterial continuous measurements of blood pressure would have been preferable in all test subjects. It would also have been interesting to measure respiration with other non-intrusive techniques such as transthoracic impedance.

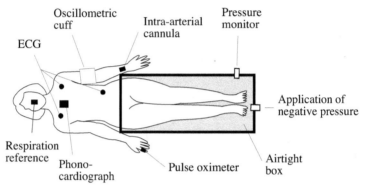

Fig. 1.7: Measurement setup for data set I.

Data set II
Contains PCG signals with various degrees of aortic stenosis present. Signals from 27 boxer dogs (15 females, 12 males, mean age 2.15 ± 2.18 years) were recorded with an electronic stethoscope (M30, Meditron AS, Oslo, Norway) and a standard 3-lead ECG (Analyzer ECG, Meditron AS, Oslo, Norway) was recorded in parallel as a time reference. For characterization purposes, all dogs underwent an echocardiographic examination. The peak aortic flow velocity, measured by continuous wave Doppler, was used as a hemodynamic reference to assess AS severity. The murmurs ranged from physiological murmurs to severe aortic stenosis murmurs (flow velocities $1.5 - 5.5$ m/s).

The dogs were divided into two groups (A and B), each of which were further divided into two subgroups of increasing stenosis severity. Group A showed no morphologic evidence of AS via 2D echocardiography and consisted of subgroup A1 ($V_{max} < 1.8$ m/s) and A2 ($V_{max} \geq 1.8$ m/s). Group B showed morphological evidence of AS on 2D echocardiography and were allocated to subgroup B1 ($V_{max} \leq 3.2$ m/s [mild AS]) and B2 ($V_{max} > 3.2$ m/s [moderate to severe AS]). The subgroup classification was based on categorization described in the veterinary medical literature [122]. Echocardiographic and auscultatory information about this data set is presented in table 1.2.

Table 1.2: Echocardiographic and auscultatory data for all dogs in data set II. The group denomination was based on peak aortic flow velocity, as outlined in the main text.

Class	A1	A2	B1	B2
Number of dogs	8	8	5	6
Degree of heart murmur (0-VI)	0–II	0–II	II–IV	III–V
Aortic flow velocity, mean ± SD (m/s)	1.65 ± 0.09	2.02 ± 0.19	2.82 ± 0.36	4.68 ± 0.57
Aortic flow velocity, range (m/s)	$1.52 - 1.73$	$1.84 - 2.41$	$2.40 - 3.20$	$4.00 - 5.50$
2D morphological aortic stenosis	No	No	Yes	Yes

Limitations: The gold standard for diagnosis of subvalvular AS in dogs is necropsy, a procedure that, for obvious reasons, was not possible to perform for research purposes. The best clinical diagnostic method available to date is echocardiography. Nevertheless, there is no single value of velocity, gradient or valve area that is able to assess AS severity alone. Of these measures, aortic flow velocity is the most reproducible and the strongest predictor of clinical outcome [175]. Further, patients with significant AS and left-sided congestive heart failure have a diminished and sometimes undetectable murmur. This important patient group is not represented in this data set.

Data set III

Contains PCG signals with various degrees of mitral insufficiency present. Signals from 77, mostly Cavalier King Charles Spaniels (CKCS), dogs (41 females, 36 males, mean age 8.60±0.34 years) were recorded with an electronic stethoscope (M30, Meditron AS, Oslo, Norway) and a standard 3-lead ECG (Analyzer ECG, Meditron AS, Oslo, Norway) was recorded in parallel as a time reference. Based on auscultation, the dogs were divided into the following murmur groups: absent (no audible heart murmur), mild (grade 1–2), moderate (grade 3–4) and severe (grade 5–6). The most commonly recruited breeds were CKCS (n=59) and Dachshund (n=5). Thirteen other breeds with one dog each were also represented in the data set.

For characterization purposes, all dogs underwent an echocardiographic examination. Assessment of mitral valve structures was conducted from the right parasternal long-axis view and the left apical four-chamber view. The same views were also used for assessing the degree of mitral regurgitation by color Doppler. Further, the left atrial to aortic root ratio (La/Ao-ratio) was quantified from a right 2-D short-axis view and M-mode measurements of the left ventricle were made. The M-mode values were used to derive the fractional shortening (FS) and the percent increase in left ventricular internal dimensions in diastole (LVIDd$_{inc}$) and in systole (LVIDs$_{inc}$) according to Cornell et al. [45]. The dogs were then classified as normal if no signs of anatomical or functional cardiac pathology could be found. Estimation of MI severity (mild, moderate and severe) was based on the obtained echocardiographic information regarding La/Ao-ratio and severity of regurgitation into the left atrium (table 1.3). More information about assessing MI in dogs can be found in Häggström et al. [100].

Limitations: Characterization of regurgitant valve lesions is among the most difficult

Table 1.3: Echocardiographic and auscultatory data for all dogs in data set III. The group denomination was based on the echocardiographic results, as outlined in the main text.

	Normal LA/Ao < 1.5 No regurgitation	Mild MI LA/Ao < 1.5 Mild regurg.	Moderate MI LA/Ao < 1.8 Moderate regurg.	Severe MI LA/Ao > 1.8 Severe regurg.
Number of dogs	5	38	17	17
HR (bpm)	103.5–167	97-121.3	93.5-135.5	115-150
LA/Ao	1.09–1.16	1.16–1.26	1.48–1.7	1.97–2.35
LVIDs (mm)	1.75–1.96	1.94–2.35	2.04–2.76	2.05–2.6
LVIDs inc (%)	-9.45–6.34	2.02–21.5	3.37–21.8	7.03–29.4
LVIDd (mm)	2.6–2.81	2.91–3.43	3.21–4.21	4.05–4.77
LVIDd inc (%)	-11.2– -4.97	-1.89–11.1	7.05–29.4	27.7–55.2
FS (%)	26.8–37.1	27.7–36.7	31.7–42.2	43.1–47.7
Auscultation	Absent	Absent–Moderate	Mild–Severe	Moderate–Severe

problems in valvular heart disease. Contributing to the difficulty of assessing mitral regurgitation is the lack of a gold standard [255]. For example, an increase in blood pressure causes an increase in the parameters used to assess MR. Here, the main parameter for MI assessment was the La/Ao-ratio which was derived from 2D echocardiography. Complementary parameters based on Doppler measurements such as the jet area, the diameter of vena contracta and the proximal isovelocity surface area (PISA) method could have been used to get a more comprehensive picture of the disease state. However, none of the Doppler parameters have been shown to be more accurate in assessing MI compared to the LA/Ao-ratio in dogs [32, 100].

Data set IV
Contains PCG signals with systolic murmurs present. Signals from 36 patients (19 male, 17 female, mean age 69 years) with probable valvular heart disease (as detected with auscultation) were included in the study (7 physiological murmurs, 23 aortic stenosis and 6 mitral insufficiency, all with native heart valves). An electronic stethoscope (theStethoscope, Meditron AS, Oslo, Norway) was used to acquire the PCG signals and a standard 3-lead ECG (Analyzer ECG, Meditron AS, Oslo, Norway) was recorded in parallel as a time reference. Both signals were digitized at 44.1 kHz with 16-bits per sample using a sound card (Analyzer, Meditron AS). PCG data were recorded successively for 15 seconds from the four traditional areas of auscultation [226]. Based on signal quality, one of the four signals was selected after visual and auditive inspection. The diagnosis and the assessment of valve lesions were based on an echocardiographic examination according to clinical routine and recommended standards [194]. The PCG signals were acquired in association with this examination.

Limitations: The severity of the disease in the AS and MI patients ranged from mild to severe, and further subdivision of these groups would have been interesting. However, the limited amount of patients in this data set prevent such groupings.

Data set V

Contains PCG signals in the presence of lung sounds. Signals from six healthy male subjects aged 28 ± 4 years were recorded with a contact accelerometer (Siemens EMT25C, Sweden), connected to a microphone amplifier (Siemens, E285E, Sweden). A standard 3-lead ECG was also recorded as a time reference (S&W, Diascope DS 521, Denmark). Both signals were digitized at 6 kHz with 12-bits per sample (National Instruments, DAQCard-700), after passing an anti-aliasing filter with a cut-off frequency of 2 kHz. The recording site was the second intercostal space along the left sternal border, and the sensor was fixed with an adhesive elastic tape. The acquisition protocol consisted of three phases: 30 s of tidal breathing, about 60 s of breathing with continuously increasing breath volumes up to vital capacity, and 10 s of breath hold (respiration rate was not controlled).

Limitations: Air flow measured with a pneumotachograph should have been acquired along with the sound signals. Controlled breathing with a predefined air flow target is essential for performance comparisons at different flow rates. Further, only healthy subjects with known cardiac (no additive sounds or murmurs) and respiratory (no crackles or wheezes) states were included in the data set.

Data set VI

Contains PCG signals with a third heart sound present (S3). Signals from ten healthy children (5 male, 5 female, mean age 10.5 years) were recorded with a contact accelerometer (Siemens, EMT 25C, Sweden) connected to a microphone amplifier (Siemens, E285E, Sweden). A standard 3-lead ECG was also recorded as a time reference (S&W, Diascope DS 521, Denmark). Both signals were digitized at 2.5 kHz with 12-bits per sample (National Instruments, DAQCard-700), after passing an anti-aliasing filter with a cut-off frequency of 1.25 kHz. The signals were recorded over the apex in a soundproof room. The sensor was fixed with a belt around the body. 30 seconds of data was acquired during breath hold, and the presence of S3 was determined by visual inspection of the recordings (an S3 occurrence was marked if a signal component with low frequency was present in a time window $120 - 200$ ms after S2).

Limitations: Ten healthy children were included in the data set since third heart sounds with high signal quality are common in this group. Patients with heart failure would have been a more appropriate study population. Another limitation is the lack of an objective and quantitative reference method for detection of S3 occurrences.

11

2

Origin of Heart Sounds and Murmurs

"The heart is of such density that fire can scarcely damage it."
Leonardo da Vinci (1452–1519)

Heart sounds and murmurs arise as a consequence of turbulent blood flow and vibrating cardiovascular structures. This chapter reviews the principles of anatomy and physiology that are necessary to understand how the cardiac sounds are related to physiological events. The electrical and mechanical operation of the healthy heart is reviewed in section 2.1 along with the most important interactions within the cardiovascular system. The coupling between the cardiac system, the vascular system and the respiratory system is very interesting since it renders continuous, non-invasive and non-intrusive monitoring of respiration and blood pressure changes possible (these particular applications will be discussed in chapter 7).

The most important parameters governing mechanical activity are blood pressure, tension in the heart or in adjacent vessels, ventricular volume, blood flow velocity and movement as well as deformation of the heart wall [234]. Many of these parameters can only be measured with sophisticated equipment. However, since the mechanical events cause vibrations that are propagated to the chest surface, information about the working status of the heart can be obtained by auscultation (section 2.3). There are basically two types of sounds originating from the heart, heart sounds and murmurs. A preliminary example showing a recorded PCG signal, containing the two normal heart sounds S1 and S2, is illustrated in figure 2.1 along with an ECG. Information about the ECG signal will be given in section 2.1.2 and the flow induced sounds giving rise to the PCG signal will be discussed in section 2.5.

Murmurs can be of both pathological or physiological origin and arise as a consequence of increased blood flow velocities in the heart. High flow velocities can be completely normal, especially amongst children, but it may also be due to a pathological narrowing in the blood's pathway. A common cause of such obstructions is valvular heart diseases, why the cause and pathophysiology of the most common valvular dysfunctions will be described in section 2.2. The concept of sounds induced by turbulence is introduced in section 2.5.2, and these ideas provide a foundation to the methodology used in upcoming chapters.

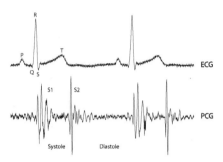

Fig. 2.1: An electrocardiogram (ECG) and a phonocardiographic (PCG) signal from a healthy person without murmurs. The ECG signal, which will be introduced in section 2.1.2, reflects electrical activity in the heart. Details about the PCG signal, here including the first heart sound (S1) and the second heart sound (S2), will be discussed in section 2.5.1.

Auscultation and phonocardiography are introduced in sections 2.3 and 2.4, together with a short survey of recording techniques. Finally, mathematical models of the two heart sounds as well as animal models of AS and MI are presented in section 2.6. The mathematical models are later used in the simulation study in chapter 4, while the animal models are used in chapter 5.

2.1 Cardiovascular anatomy and physiology

The cardiovascular system is designed to establish and maintain a mean systemic arterial pressure sufficient to transport nutrients, oxygen and waste products to and from the cells, while preserving regulatory flexibility, minimizing cardiac work and stabilizing body temperature and pH to maintain homeostasis [119]. The main components of the cardiovascular system are the heart, the blood, and the blood vessels.

The primary task of the heart is to serve as a pump propelling blood around the circulatory system. When the heart contracts, blood is forced through the valves. First from the atria to the ventricles and then from the ventricles out through the body, see figure 2.2. There are four heart chambers, the right and left atria and the right and left ventricles. From a simplistic[1] point of view, the two atria act as collecting reservoirs for blood returning to the heart while the two ventricles act as pumps ejecting blood out through the body. The pumping action of the heart is divided into two phases; systole when the ventricles contract and ejects blood from the heart, and diastole, when the ventricles are relaxed and the heart is filled with blood. Four valves prevent the blood from flowing backwards; the atrioventricular valves (the mitral and tricuspid valve) prevent blood from flowing

---

[1]The contraction of the heart is actually very intriguing, where the pumping action is a complex 3D motion involving effects such as valve plane motion and wall thickening.

14

back from the ventricles to the atria and the semilunar valves (aortic and pulmonary valves) prevent blood from flowing back towards the ventricles once being pumped into the aorta and the pulmonary artery, respectively. Deoxygenated blood from the body enters the right atrium, passes into the right ventricle and is ejected out through the pulmonary artery on its way to the lungs. Oxygenated blood from the lungs re-enter the heart in the left atrium, passes into the left ventricle and is then ejected out through the body.

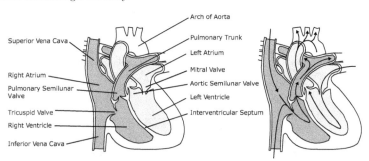

Fig. 2.2: Anatomy of the heart (left figure) and the blood flow pathways through left and right side of the heart (right figure).

2.1.1 The heart valves

The atria are separated from the ventricles by the fibrous skeleton of the heart [119]. There is one fibrous ring around each of the four valves, but the rings are fused together into a single fibrous framework. The skeleton has several physiological functions; it provides a foundation to which the valves and the great arteries attach, it prevents overstretching of the valves as blood passes through them and it electrically isolates the atria from the ventricles[2] (see also section 2.1.2). All four heart valves have flaps, called leaflets or cusps, which open to let the blood flow through and close to prevent blood from flowing backwards. The valves and their leaflets are illustrated in figure 2.3.

The mitral and tricuspid valve leaflets are connected via the chordae tendineae and papillary muscles to the ventricular wall. The papillary muscles contract at the same time as the ventricles contract, thus pulling the chordae tendineae downwards and preventing the valve leaflets from everting into the atria. The semilunar valves both have three cusps consisting of connective tissue reinforced by fibers. These valves do not have chordae tendineae, instead the shape of the cusps prevent any form of prolapse.

---

[2]The only electrical conduction link between the atria and the ventricles goes through the atrioventricular bundle which penetrates the fibrous skeleton in a location between the mitral, aortic and tricuspid valves [119].

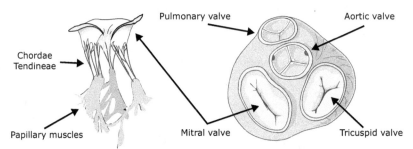

Fig. 2.3: Illustration of the mitral valve and its associated chordae tendineae and papillary muscles (left) and the heart valves and the fibrous rings surrounding each valve (right).

2.1.2 The cardiac electrical system

Cardiac muscle cells can possess at least four properties: *automaticity* (the ability to initiate an electrical impulse), *conductivity* (the ability to conduct electrical impulses), *contractility* (the ability to shorten and do work) and *lusitropy* (the ability to relax) [25]. Cells in different areas of the heart are specialized to perform different tasks; all cells possess the conductivity property, the working cells are mainly able to contract and relax while the cells governing the electric systems are adapted to automaticity and conductivity. The pumping action of the heart is synchronized by *pacemaker cells*, concentrated in the sinoatrial node (located in the right atrium), the atrioventricular node (located in the wall between the atria) and in the His-Purkinje system (starting in the atrioventricular node and spreading over the ventricles), see figure 2.4.

An action potential generated in the sinoatrial node (which normally controls the heart rate) will spread through the atria and initiate atrial contraction. The atria are electrically isolated from the ventricles, connected only via the atrioventricular node which briefly delays the signal. The delay in the transmission allows the atria to empty before the ventricles contract. The distal part of the atrioventricular node is referred to as the *Bundle of His*. The Bundle of His splits into two branches, the left bundle branch and the right bundle branch, activating the left and the right ventricle, respectively. The action potential spreads very quickly through the ventricle due to the fast His-Purkinje cells, causing almost immediate synchronous excitation of the entire ventricular wall [217].

The electrocardiogram (ECG)
Cardiac action potentials are conducted to the body surface, where they can be measured as an electrical potential that varies with the current flow through the heart. Action potentials associated with different cardiac regions are illustrated in figure 2.4 along with a typical ECG waveform measured from the body surface. The ECG can be seen as a projection of a dominant vector (represented by the summation in time and space of the action potentials from each muscle cell) onto a lead vector, whose direction is defined by the position of the measurement electrodes

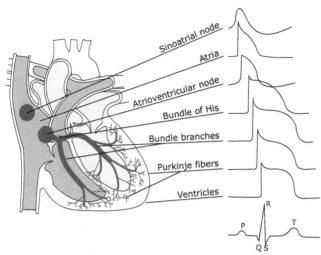

Fig. 2.4: Morphology and timing of action potentials from different regions of the heart are illustrated in the right-hand side of the figure. Also illustrated is the related ECG signal as measured on the body surface. Redrawn from Sörnmo and Laguna [217].

in relation to the heart [217]. The ECG describes the different electrical phases of the heart, where depolarization of the atria gives rise to the P-wave, depolarization of the ventricles combined with repolarization of the atria results in the QRS-complex and repolarization of the ventricles results in the T-wave.

2.1.3 The cardiac cycle and the pressure-volume loop

The blood pressure within a chamber increases as the heart contracts, generating a flow from higher pressure areas towards lower pressure areas. The work diagram of the heart, illustrated in figure 2.5 for the left ventricle, is referred to as a pressure-volume (PV) loop [119]. The following discussion applies to the left side of the heart, but the key concepts are similar for the right side.

When left atrial pressure exceeds the pressure in the left ventricle, the mitral valve opens (A) and the atrium empties into the ventricle (*filling*). During the rapid filling phase, venous blood from the lungs enters the atrium, and as the pressure gradient between the atrium and the ventricle levels out (reduced filling phase), a final volume of blood is forced into the ventricle by atrial contraction. When tension develops in the ventricular wall, increased intraventricular pressure will force the mitral valve to shut (B). The pressure stretching the ventricle at this moment is called *preload*. The amount of pressure exerted is determined by the duration of ventricular diastole together with the venous pressure. Within limits, the more the heart is stretched during diastole, the more vigorous the contraction will be in systole. Since the heart is contracting while all valves are closed, ventricular pressure will increase whereas the volume remains unchanged (*isovolumic contraction*). The first heart

17

sound originates from events related to the closing of the mitral valve (B) and the opening of the aortic valve (C). The ventricular pressure required to open the aortic valve is called *afterload*, a parameter which, consequently, is affected by arterial blood pressure.

As blood is *ejected* from the heart, ventricular pressure decreases, and when it falls below the aortic pressure, the aortic valve closes again (D). In association with valve closure, S2 is heard. The end-systolic pressure-volume ratio is a clinical measure of cardiac muscle performance referred to as *myocardial contractility*. Again all valves are closed, but this time the pressure will decrease while the volume remains unchanged. This phase, called *isovolumetric relaxation*, will complete the loop and start a new heart cycle.

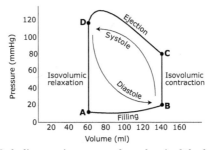

Fig. 2.5: Work diagram (pressure-volume loop) of the left ventricle.

The PV-loop illustrates the changing pressures and flows within the heart, however, it has no time scale. Wiggers diagram, see figure 2.6, demonstrates the temporal correlations between electrical and mechanical events in the left side of the heart over one cardiac cycle [119]. The electrical R-wave, representing ventricular depolarization, precedes the beginning of ventricular contraction. The ventricular contraction causes a rapid rise in the left ventricular pressure. As soon as the ventricular pressure exceeds the atrial pressure, the mitral valve closes (B in the PV-loop). This is when S1 is heard. When the ventricular pressure exceeds the aortic pressure, the aortic valve opens (C in the PV-loop), and the blood flows from the ventricle to the aorta. At the end of blood ejection, the pressure in the ventricle falls below the aortic pressure, and the aortic valve closes (D in the PV-loop), giving rise to S2. The pressure in the ventricle drops steeply, and when it falls below the atrial pressure, the mitral valve opens (A in the PV-loop), and the rapid filling phase begins. The rapid filling phase might cause an impact sound, the third heart sound (S3), when blood collides with the ventricular wall. Similarly, atrial systole may also produce an audible forth heart sound (S4). S3 and S4 will be described more carefully in section 2.5.

2.1.4 Coupling in the cardiovascular system

As stated before, the main task of the cardiovascular system is to efficiently maintain an arterial pressure which is high enough to meet the flow demands of the body's

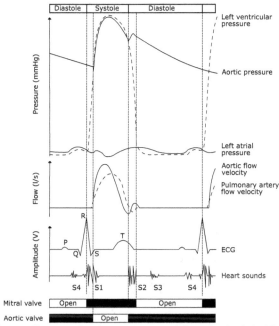

Fig. 2.6: Wiggers diagram, showing pressures and flows in the left side of the heart over one heart cycle and how they relate to electrical (ECG) and mechanical (PCG) activity.

tissues. Blood pressure refers to the force exerted by circulating blood on the walls of blood vessels, and is directly determined by the arterial blood volume and arterial compliance [25]. These physical factors are in turn affected primarily by cardiac output and peripheral vessel resistance (whose product approximately equals mean arterial pressure).

Cardiac output is defined as the heart rate times the stroke volume. The *cardiac electrical system* is the main rate controller, whose task is to synchronize the cardiac mechanical system. The most important regulators of heart rate are the *autonomous nervous system* (sympathetic activity increases heart rate while parasympathetic activity decreases heart rate) and *the hormonal system* [25].

The *cardiac mechanical system* is mainly regulated by the three factors controlling stroke volume: preload, afterload and myocardial contractility (see section 2.1.3). Heart rate and contractility are strict cardiac factors while preload and afterload depend on both cardiac and vascular factors. These latter two provide a functional coupling between the heart and the blood vessels since both preload and afterload are important determinants of cardiac output. However, at the same time, they are also determined by cardiac output [25].

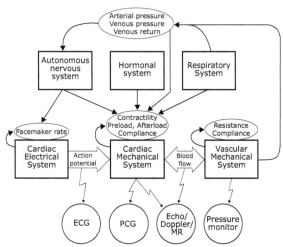

Fig. 2.7: Diagram surveying different interactions between the systems involved in cardiac activity along with various measurable signals. The illustration should not be considered complete, it rather functions as a facilitator of the main text. The abbreviated measurable signals at the bottom are the electrocardiogram (ECG), phonocardiogram (PCG), echocardiogram (ECG), Doppler ultrasound (Doppler)and magnetic resonance imaging (MR).

The *respiratory system* causes periodic changes in the intra-thoracic pressure, effecting blood flow, venous pressure and venous return [25]. Amongst others, changes in diastolic filling of the heart lead to rhythmic variations in cardiac output (the heart rate is increased during inspiration and decreased during expiration, a phenomenon called respiratory sinus arrhythmia). A schematic illustration of interconnections in the cardiovascular system is given in figure 2.7.

In physics, two systems are coupled if they are interacting with each other. The cardiovascular system is interconnected through many different feedback control loops, why coupling is an innate and natural property of the system. Unfortunately, since most components are interdependent on each other, it is very difficult to elucidate these interactions. In fact, most of these interconnections are not understood. Some possible (and probable) interactions are the ones illustrated in figure 2.7.

From figure 2.7, it can also be seen that the vascular mechanical system is affected by both the respiratory system and the cardiac system. These interactions can be used to gain information about physiological parameters that are not directly measured. For example, in chapter 7, information gained from the ECG and the PCG are utilized to track blood pressure changes and to monitor respiration via cardiac time intervals.

2.1.5 Fractal physiology

It has been suggested that the regulation of the heart possesses fractal characteristics [79]. A fractal can be described in at least three contexts: geometrical, temporal and statistical. Common for the three is that the object/signal should be self-similar. This means that the fractal consists of subunits that resemble the larger scale shape, or, similarly, when zooming into a fractal you end up with something that looks like what you started out with. Examples of cardiac anatomical structures that appear self-similar are the coronary arterial and venous trees, the chordae tendineae and the His-Purkinje network. These are all examples of geometrical fractals. A modern, and somewhat controversial, hypothesis is that the regulation of heart rate is also a fractal process. Creating a time series of interbeat intervals, it can be shown that the fluctuations in the series have a broadband spectrum following a 1/f-distribution [79]. Whether this hypothesis of fractal physiology is valid remains to be seen, but it is an interesting approach in the pursuit of an explanation of cardiovascular control.

2.2 Valvular heart diseases

Valvular heart diseases are more common in the mitral and aortic valves since the left side of the heart sustains higher pressures and greater workloads. There are two major problems that may compromise the functionality of the valves, stenosis and insufficiency [174]. In *stenosis* the leaflets become rigid, thickened or fused together, reducing the opening through which the blood passes from one chamber to another. The obstructed flow gives rise to an accumulation of blood in the chamber, forcing the heart to work harder in order to pump the blood. In *insufficiency* (or *regurgitation*) the valves fail to close properly why a portion of the ejected blood flows backward. For example, if the mitral valve is unable to close properly, some of the blood will leak back into the left atrium during systole.

Valvular stenosis and insufficiency gradually wear out the heart. At first, the heart muscle thickens (hypertrophy) and the heart enlarges (dilatation), thus compensating for the extra workload and allowing the heart to supply an adequate amount of blood to the body. Over time, the overdeveloped heart muscle may lead to a functional degradation and heart failure.

Aortic stenosis (AS) is an obstruction between the left ventricle and the aorta, see figure 2.8. The obstruction may be in the valve (valvular), above the valve (supravalvular) or below the valve (subvalvular). The most common causes are congenital abnormality, rheumatic fever, or calcific degeneration or deposits of calcium on the valve. In the presence of an obstruction, a pressure gradient develops between the left ventricle and the ascending aorta. As a response to the increased left ventricular pressure, hypertrophy is developed. Since left ventricular hypertrophy offers increased resistance to filling, preload is elevated (through strong atrial contractions). Eventually, the increased left atrial pressure produces pulmonary edema, leading to increased pressures in the right side of the heart, increased systemic venous pressure and peripheral edema [174].

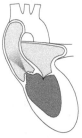 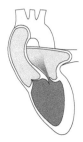

Aortic valve stenosis   Mitral insufficiency

Fig. 2.8: Schematic illustration of the left side of the heart in the presence of AS (left) and MI (right). In AS, the passageway to aorta is narrowed, causing turbulent flow distal to the valves. Hypertrophy is often seen as a consequence to the increased flow resistance. In MI, the mitral valve is unable to close completely, causing blood to leak back into the left atrium during systole.

Aortic insufficiency refers to an incompetent aortic valve allowing blood to flow back into the left ventricle during diastole when the ejection is complete. In its acute form, aortic regurgitation usually occurs as a result of infective endocarditis that destroys the valve's leaflets. The chronic form, which is more common, is usually a consequence of widening of the aorta in the region where it connects to the valve. In either case, the constant leaking of blood results in increased left ventricular diastolic pressure, increased left atrial pressure and eventually heart failure and pulmonary edema [174].

Mitral stenosis is a narrowing or blockage of the mitral valve, often as a result of rheumatic fever. The narrowed valve causes blood to back up in the left atrium instead of flowing into the left ventricle and results in an increase in the pressure in the left atrium. This pressure is transmitted back through the pulmonary veins, causing pulmonary edema and consequent problems in the right side of the heart [174].

Mitral insufficiency (MI) is an abnormal leaking of blood from the left ventricle into the left atrium of the heart, see figure 2.8. The most common causes are myxomatous degeneration of the valve, annulus dilatation, dysfunction of the papillary muscles or rupture of the chordae tendineae. The amount of blood that flows back into the atrium is called a regurgitant volume. The regurgitant volume depends on three factors: the area of the leaking orifice, the pressure gradient between the chambers and the regurgitant duration. Since blood is ejected into the left atrium instead of out through the aorta, the forward stroke volume decreases. In response, the heart compensates by increasing the total stroke volume and the heart rate, and by eccentric hypertrophy. The atrium will increase its force of contraction in order to maintain ventricular filling. The consequent increase in atrial pressure may lead to pulmonary congestion and edema [174].

Tricuspid and pulmonic stenosis and regurgitation only account for a small amount of the valve diseases and is most often secondary to disease in the left side of the heart. Abnormalities of the tricuspid valve are generally caused by rheumatic fever or metabolic abnormalities. Edema and fatigue are the major symptoms produced by tricuspid valve dysfunction. Pulmonary valve dysfunction is also rare and is primarily due to congenital defects.

The causes of heart valve damage vary depending on the type of disease, but may include [52]:

- *Rheumatic Fever:* an inflammatory condition that often starts with strep throat or scarlet fever. Though the disease is rarely fatal during the acute stage, it may lead to rheumatic valvular disease, a chronic and progressive condition that causes cardiac disability or death many years after the initial event [174]. The damage is not caused by the bacteria themselves, but by an autoimmune response - a process in which the body mistakenly begins to damage its own tissues.

- *Infective Endocarditis:* a disease caused by microbial infection of the endothelial lining of the heart [174]. The infection can cause vegetations on the heart valves, which sometimes conjures new or altered heart murmurs, particularly murmurs suggestive of valvular regurgitation [226].

- *Myxomatous degeneration:* a pathological weakening, mainly affecting the mitral valve. This dysfunction stems from a series of metabolic changes, causing the valve's tissue to lose its elasticity while becoming weak and covered by deposits.

- *Calcific degeneration:* a hardening formed by deposits of calcium salts on the valve. This type of tissue degeneration usually causes AS, a narrowing of the aortic valve [174].

- *Congenital anomalies:* abnormal structures in the heart. The most common congenital valve defect is bicuspid aortic valves (two leaflets instead of three). Although not a valvular disease, septal defects (an abnormal passage between the left and the right side of the heart) should also be mentioned since they are also congenital anomalies which gives rise to murmurs. Ventricular septal defect is generally considered to be the most common type of malformation, accounting for 28% of all congenital heart defects [174].

Other causes include heart valve diseases that result from other heart diseases, particularly coronary artery disease or myocardial infarction. These conditions can cause injury to one of the papillary muscles that support the valves, or annulus dilatation, so that the valve does not close properly.

2.3 Auscultation and phonocardiography

The technique of deciphering the sounds from the body based on their intensity, frequency, duration, number and quality is called auscultation [254]. The acoustical signal is affected by a chain of transfer functions before the physician's actual decision-making process starts. The signal transmitted from the sound source is propagated through the human body, where the sound waves are both reflected and

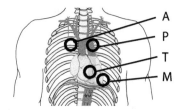

Fig. 2.9: The traditional auscultatory areas on the chest (M refers to the mitral area, T the tricuspid area, P the pulmonic area, and A the aortic area).

absorbed. The most compressible tissues such as lung tissue and fat contribute most to the absorption. Low frequencies are less attenuated compared to high frequencies, but the high frequencies are easier to perceive (see figure 2.11 and the accompanying text in section 2.5). The consequences of the attenuation are therefore hard to predict. To reduce the effect of thoracic damping, certain areas of cardiac auscultation have been defined. In these locations, the sound is transmitted through solid tissues or through a minimal thickness of lung tissue. The traditional areas of auscultation (figure 2.9), where the radiated sound intensity from each of the four heart valves is maximized, are defined as [226]:

- Mitral area: The cardiac apex.
- Tricuspid area: The fourth and fifth intercostal space along the left sternal border.
- Aortic area: The second intercostal space along the right sternal border.
- Pulmonic area: The second intercostal space along the left sternal border.

Even though the definition of these areas came to life long before much understanding of the physiology of the heart was available, they remain good starting positions. Revised areas of auscultation, allowing more degrees of freedom, have however been adopted [226].

Auscultation is usually performed with a stethoscope (figure 1.1), which constitutes the second transfer function affecting the sound signal. A basic stethoscope consists of three components: the earpieces, the tubing and the chest piece [226]. The chest piece looks like a funnel, either covered by a membrane (diaphragm mode) or without a membrane (bell mode). A wider chest piece conveys better signal transfers, but the size is practically limited by the curvature of the body. It is important that the chest piece fits tightly against the body because air leakage heavily distorts and weakens the signal. The bell is used to pick up low frequency sounds such as S3 and S4, whereas the diaphragm is used to pick up high frequency sounds such as lung sounds and certain murmurs. From the chest piece the sound is propagated through the tubing to the ear pieces. Due to the standing wave phenomenon, amplification peaks arise when the length of the tuning coincide with the quarter wavelength of the sounds. Binaural stethoscopes, where the tubing divides in two, gives rise to very complicated resonance patterns. The electronic stethoscope was introduced to avoid the resonances introduced by the tubing. The bell and the diaphragm are then replaced by a broad-band acoustic sensor and an amplifier, whereas the tubing and the ear pieces are replaced by wires and head phones. The single most important problem with electronic stethoscopes is that the physician does not recognize what they hear when the resonances no longer alter the sounds.

The third and last transfer function which affects the sound is the physicians' auditory system. As will be mentioned in section 2.5, human hearing is nonlinear and frequency dependent. Further, sound reception deteriorates with age. Fortunately this age discrepancy mainly affects high frequencies above the bioacoustical range.

2.3.1 Terminology for describing cardiac sounds

Of the two normal heart sounds, S1 is louder, longer and lower pitched compared to S2. While S1 and S2 are referred to as tones, murmurs are characterized by a sound most easily described as "noise-like". During auscultation, murmurs are described by a number of factors: timing in the cardiac cycle, intensity on a scale of I-VI, shape, frequency, point of maximal intensity and radiation. A grade I murmur is very faint and heard only with special effort while grade VI is extremely loud and accompanied by a palpable thrill. When the intensity of systolic murmurs is crescendo-decrescendo shaped and ends before one or both of the components of S2, it is assumed to be an ejection murmur. Murmurs due to backward flow across the atrioventricular valves are of even intensity throughout systole and reach one or both components of S2. If the regurgitant systolic murmur starts with S1 it is called holosystolic and if it begins in mid or late systole it is called a late systolic regurgitant murmur. Besides murmurs, ejection clicks might also be heard in systole. They are often caused by abnormalities in the pulmonary or aortic valves. Different murmurs, snaps, knocks and plops can also be heard in diastole, but such diastolic sounds are beyond the scope of this book. [226]

2.3.2 Phonocardiography (PCG)

A graphical representation of the waveform of cardiac sounds is called a phonocardiogram, and the technique used to capture the sound signal is referred to as phonocardiography. Examples of PCG signals have already been shown in chapter 1 as well as in figures 2.1 and 2.6. This technique allows a visual interpretation of the cardiac sounds, thus allowing thorough investigation of temporal dependencies between mechanical processes of the heart and the sounds produced. Today, PCG is mainly used for teaching and training purposes [234], but since new electronic stethoscopes make the recording procedure much easier, PCG might make a comeback in clinical practise.

2.4 Acquisition of PCG signals

The audio recording chain involves a sequence of transformations of the signal: a sensor to convert sound or vibrations to electricity, a pre-amplifier to amplify the signal, a prefilter to avoid aliasing and an analogue to digital converter to convert the signal to digital form. In addition, the chain can be complemented with an analysis step and an information presentation step.

Sensors
Microphones and accelerometers are the natural choice of sensor when recording sound. These sensors have a high-frequency response that is quite adequate for body sounds. Rather, it is the low-frequency region that might cause problems [169]. The microphone is an air coupled sensor that measures pressure waves induced by chest-wall movements while accelerometers are contact sensors which directly measure chest-wall movements. For recording of body sounds, both kinds can be used. More precisely, condenser microphones and piezoelectric accelerometers have been recommended [231].

Electronic stethoscopes make use of sensors specially designed for cardiac sounds. Compared to classical stethoscopes, electronic stethoscopes try to make heart and lung sounds more clearly audible by using different filters and amplifiers. Some also allow storage and the possibility to connect the stethoscope to a computer for further analysis of the recorded sounds. The leading suppliers of electronic stethoscopes are Cardionics, Thinklabs, Meditron (Welch-Allyn) and 3M (Littmann). Thinklabs uses a novel electronic diaphragm detection system to directly convert sounds into electronic signals. Welch-Allyn Meditron uses a piezo-electric sensor on a metal shaft inside the chest piece, while 3M and Cardionics use conventional microphones. More recently, ambient noise filtering has become available in electronic stethoscopes.

In the data sets used in this book, two different sensors have been used; the Siemens Elema EMT25C contact accelerometer and electronic stethoscopes from Welch-Allyn Meditron (M30 or theStethoscope, Meditron ASA, Oslo, Norway).

Pre-processing, digitalization and storage
The preamplifier amplifies the low level transducer signals to line level. By doing this, the full range of the analogue to digital converter is used, thus minimizing quantization errors. In the digitalization of signals, aliasing will occur unless the Nyquist-Shannon sampling theorem is fulfilled.

In the data sets using EMT25C, a custom-built replica of a PCG amplifier (Siemens Elema E285E) was used. This amplifier included a low-pass filter with a cut-off frequency of 2 kHz. The signal was digitized with 12-bits per sample using analogue to digital converters from National Instruments. Acquisition of the data was conducted in a Labview-application (National Instruments, Austin, Texas, US) after which the data were stored on a personal computer.

For the electronic stethoscope, the associated acquisition equipment and software were used (Analyzer, Meditron ASA, Oslo, Norway). According to the manufacturer, the digital recordings are stored without pre-filtering. An excessive sampling frequency of 44.1 kHz was thus used to avoid aliasing and with the idea of post-filtering in mind. The signals were stored in a database on a personal computer.

A comparison of different sensors and sensor designs is out of the scope of this book. However, this is an important matter. The developed signal processing methodology might be affected by the frequency response of the sensors, and if this is the case, these issues must be elucidated. It is however unlikely that the sensor characteristics influence the results to any greater extent. For example, the heart sound localization approaches that will be described in chapter 4 were not noticeably affected by the two different sensors used to collect the test signals (EMT25C and Meditron M30). Considering that the frequency characteristics of these two sensors are very different (M30 has a nearly linear frequency response in the full audible range while EMT25C attenuates frequencies below 100 Hz and above 1 kHz), the developed methods seem quite robust when it comes to the choice of sensor characteristics. Nonetheless, this issue should be investigated further. Comparisons of different bioacoustic sensors has previously been performed by Grenier et al. [85] and Kraman et al. [127].

2.5 Flow-induced sound and vibrations

Sounds are generated by vibrating objects and propagate as waves of alternating pressures. The vibrating source sets particles in motion, and if the sound is a pure tone, the individual particle moves back and forth with the frequency of that tone. Each particle is thus moving around its resting point, but as it pushes nearby particles they are also set in motion and this chain effect results in areas of compression and rarefaction. The alternating areas of compression and rarefaction constitute a pressure wave that moves away from the sound source, see figure 2.10. These pressure variations can be detected via the mechanical effect they exert on a membrane (the diaphragm of a stethoscope, the tympanic membrane in the ear etc.). If the sound source vibrates in a more irregular manner, the resulting sound wave will be more complex. Usually, sound is described by its intensity, duration and frequency [31]. If the sound is nonstationary (see section 3.6), these variables have to be analyzed as a function of time to give relevant information.

Frequency is a physical entity, and what humans perceive as frequency is called pitch (unit *mel*). The two are closely related, but the relationship is not linear. Up to 1 kHz, the measured frequency and the perceived pitch are fairly the same. Above 1 kHz, a larger increase in frequency is required to create an equal perceived change in pitch. For example, if you are listening to a 2 kHz tone which suddenly changes frequency to 4 kHz, you will not perceive a doubling in frequency, but merely an increase by a factor of about 1.5. This is due to the human auditory system which is optimized to have high accuracy in the frequency range below 1 kHz (speech).

Intensity is determined by the amplitude of the vibrations, the distance the wave must travel and the medium through which it travels. Similar to frequency, intensity also has a perceived correspondence, named loudness (unit phon). Intensity and loudness are not linearly related, and figure 2.11 shows curves of equal loudness at different frequencies. For example, a frequency shift from 50 Hz to 30 Hz requires

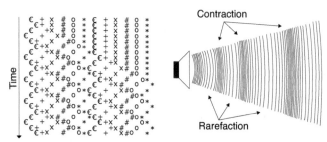

Fig. 2.10: The left figure is a schematic drawing of twelve particles in simple harmonic motion at twenty-two moments in time. The sound source is located on the left side and the pressure wave, indicated by clustering of three adjacent particles, moves from left to right. Note that each particle moves relatively little around a rest position. The traveling wave phenomenon is also illustrated in the right figure, note the regions of compression and rarefaction that are present in both subplots.

the sound to be amplified with about 10 dB to be perceived as equally loud. This phenomenon has great impact on auscultation since heart sounds are of very low frequency.

2.5.1 Heart sounds

The relationship between blood volumes, pressures and flows within the heart determines the opening and closing of the heart valves. Normal heart sounds occur during the closure of the valves, but how they are actually generated is still debated. The *valvular theory* states that heart sounds emanate from a point source located near the valves, and that the valves are the generator of all the ensuing vibrations [214]. One reason for the popularity of this theory in the clinical community is the correlation between valve vibrations as seen with echocardiography or cinematography and the occurrence of the sound [214]. However, no single structure such as a

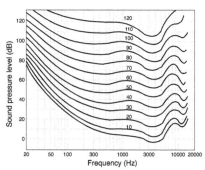

Fig. 2.11: Loudness level contours derived by Fletcher and Munson. Each curve represents a sound which is perceived to have equal loudness for all frequencies. The loudness in phons is indicated on each curve. Redrawn from Fletcher and Munson [67].

heart valve can vibrate independently without affecting the blood [202]. Blood is an incompressible fluid, so motion in one cardiac structure will quickly propagate to neighboring structures. This observation led to the *cardiohemic theory*, stating that the heart and the blood represent an interdependent system that vibrates as a whole [214]. A combination of the valvular and the cardiohemic theory, suggesting that intracardiac PCGs result from individual cardiac structures (valvular theory) while thoracic PCGs result from the mixing of several sources (cardiohemic theory), has also been suggested [54].

S1 is heard in relation to the closing of the atrioventricular valves, and is believed to include four major components [202], see figure 2.12. The initial vibrations occur when the first contraction of the ventricles accelerate blood towards the atria, just before closure of the atrioventricular valves. The second component is caused by the momentum of the moving blood as it overstretches the atrioventricular valves and recoils back towards the ventricles. The third component involves oscillation of blood between the root of the aorta (and the pulmonary artery) and the ventricular walls, and the fourth component represents the vibrations caused by turbulence in the ejected blood flowing out through aorta. Even though S1 is a composite sound arising due to events in both the right and the left side of the heart, activities from the higher pressurized left side will probably dominate the sound.

S2 signals the end of systole and the beginning of diastole, and is heard at the time of the closing of the aortic and pulmonary valves. S2 contains two components, one

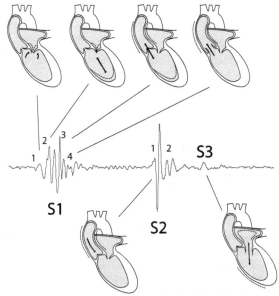

Fig. 2.12: Schematic drawing illustrating the underlying physiological causes of S1, S2 and S3. Only the left side of the heart is shown. Image redrawn after Rushmer [202].

originating from aortic valve closure and the other from pulmonary valve closure. These two coincide with the ending of left and right ventricular ejection. Since right ventricular ejection ends after left ventricular ejection, the pulmonary sound component occurs slightly after the aortic sound component. The splitting between the two components increases during inspiration because blood-return to the right heart increases, vascular capacitance of the pulmonary bed increases and blood return to the left side of the heart decreases [226]. The opposite occurs during expiration, placing the two components tightly together. S2 is probably the result of the momentum of moving blood as it overstretches the valve cusps, recoils, and initiate oscillations in both the ventricular cavities and in the arteries [202]. This causes the entire heart to move away from the arteries. The resulting vibrations, while being triggered by the valves, are also very dependent on the properties of the heart muscle.

There are also a third and a fourth heart sound (S3 and S4), both connected to the diastolic filling period. The rapid filling phase starts with the opening of the atrioventricular valves. Most investigators attribute S3 to the energy released with the sudden deceleration of blood that enters the left ventricle throughout this period [158]. A fourth heart sound may occur during atrial systole when a final volume of blood is forced into the ventricles. If the ventricles are stiff, the force of the entering blood is more vigorous, resulting in an impact sound in late diastole [226]. S3 and S4 are perhaps the best examples that heart sounds do not radiate from the valves but from vibrations in the cardiohemic system [214].

2.5.2 Murmurs and bruits

While heart sounds arise due to vibrations from acceleration and deceleration of blood and other structures in the heart, murmurs or bruits are the result of turbulence developing in rapidly flowing blood[3]. This means that a murmur can arise in a healthy heart if the blood is flowing faster than usual or if an increased amount of blood is flowing through the system. These murmurs are called innocent, normal, functional or physiological since they are completely harmless. There are mainly five factors involved in murmur production [226]:

- High rates of flow through the valves.
- Flow through a constricted valve (stenosis).
- Backward flow through an incompetent valve (insufficiency or regurgitation).
- Abnormal shunts between the left and right side of the heart (septal defects).
- Decreased blood viscosity.

The hemodynamic principles are essentially the same regardless if turbulence is produced in a vascular stenosis, a valvular stenosis or a valvular insufficiency [170]. Flow through an obstructed tube is thus a suitable model for the theoretical survey in this section.

---

[3]The term murmur is preferred when the turbulence originates from the heart (e.g. aortic valve stenosis) while the term bruit is used when the turbulence originates from a vessel (e.g. arterial stenosis).

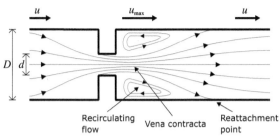

Fig. 2.13: Streamlines of flow through and distal to an orifice stenosis. The fluid flow contracts in the entrance region and reaches a minimal area in vena contracta. Image redrawn after Ask et al. [19].

Stenoses can produce large changes in local velocity due to the law of mass conservation. The reduced area at the obstructed site causes an increased flow velocity and a contraction of the fluid in the entrance region, thus creating a jet through the stenosis, see figure 2.13. Distal to the obstruction, instabilities will arise in the shear layer between the jet and surrounding fluids, introducing vortices and turbulent flow [19]. The flow regime can be described by the Reynolds number, R, which is defined as the ratio of inertial forces (ρu) to viscous forces (η/D), see equation 2.1 where ρ is the density of the fluid, D is the characteristic length[4], u is the mean fluid velocity and η is the viscosity of the fluid.

$$R = \frac{\rho D u}{\eta} \qquad (2.1)$$

Laminar flow is characterized by smooth (streamlined) fluid motion and occurs at low Reynolds numbers where viscous forces are dominant. If the flow contains random eddies, vortices and other random flow fluctuations it is called turbulent. Turbulent flow is seen at high Reynolds numbers where inertial forces are dominating. The border-line between laminar and turbulent flows is characterized by a critical Reynolds number. The transition is however not immediate. Partly turbulent flows, with time-dependent and complicated flow patterns, usually appear well before full turbulence is developed [28]. When the transition occurs depend on geometrical parameters. For example, in a long cylindrical tube, the characteristic length in equation 2.1 equals the diameter of the tube and the critical Reynolds number is typically taken as 2300[5].

At normal velocities in the cardiovascular system, the Reynolds number is low and the flow is nearly laminar. However, in the presence of obstructions such as arterial stenoses, turbulence develops at Reynolds numbers well below the traditional value of 2300. In the presence of a stenosis, the characteristic length is typically chosen as

---

[4]The characteristic length is the diameter of the largest vortices in the flow.

[5]In tubes with very smooth surfaces the critical Reynolds number can be as high as 40000. For blood vessels, the critical number is often estimated to about 2000. It is however possible that turbulence is present in unobstructed arteries for Reynolds numbers as low as $800 - 1200$ [28].

the ratio between the diameter or the length of the obstruction and the unobstructed tube area. In practise, the critical Reynolds number depends on both the geometry of the obstruction and the frequency of the pulsatile blood flow [251]. Typically, the critical value decreases with the ratio between the obstructed orifice area and the unobstructed tube area.

Turbulent flow consists of velocity fluctuations that are superimposed on the main velocity, thus inducing pressure fluctuations. These pressure fluctuations affect the vessel wall and cause vibrations in the acoustical frequency range [19]. The wall pressure amplitude reaches a maximum at the reattachment point of the jet [146], see figure 2.13, where the pressure fluctuations are mainly caused by vortices shed from the jet area [3]. At this location, the distribution of vortex sizes contains information about the diameter of the jet area, why the spectrum of the fluctuations is related to the severity of the stenosis [203]. This relation has been manifested through a Strouhal number [227] as defined in equation 2.2, where f_b is a break frequency, d is the diameter of the stenotic orifice and u_{max} is the flow velocity of the jet.

$$S = \frac{f_b d}{u_{max}} \tag{2.2}$$

The relationship between break frequency, flow velocity and lumen diameter has been found valid over a wide range of values [159]. However, the Strouhal number requires that the recorded signal is acquired close to the obstruction site. Further downstream, information about the initial conditions of the jet is lost [3]. Also, since the break frequency varies with the pulsatile and unknown flow velocity [253], the Strouhal number becomes rather difficult to apply in a clinical situation.

Kolmogorov[6] suggested that large low frequency vortices are generated at the onset of turbulence [126]. With increasing flow velocity, these large vortices pass on their energy to faster but smaller-sized vortices in a cascade of ever smaller sizes and ever higher frequencies until the smallest vortices finally vanish and turn into heat by dissipation. The size of the largest vortices is set by the overall geometry of the flow while the smallest scales are set by the Reynolds number. The spectrum of eddies, plotted as the turbulent energy contained in particular sizes of eddies versus the eddy frequency, can be described in terms of regions, see figure 2.14. In order of decreasing vortex size these regions consist of [170]:

I. Large permanent eddies (slope 0).

II. Energy containing eddies (slope -1).

III. Kolmogorov inertial, smaller size eddies (slope -5/3).

IV. Kolmogorov microscale eddies (slope -7).

---

[6]In fact, since Kolmogorov's (or actually Landau's [130]) route to turbulence has not been observed experimentally, it is now considered incorrect [216]. Alternative accounts for the onset of turbulence have been suggested, see chapter 5.

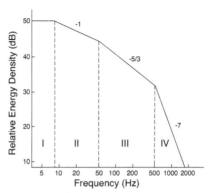

Fig. 2.14: Turbulent energy density spectrum described in terms of regions I-IV. See the text for details. Figure redrawn from Nygaard et al. [170].

In stenotic tube flow, a similar but somewhat different phenomena occurs [26]. Momentum causes the jet to persist for some time before diverging and reattaching to the vessel wall. In the separated flow region that arises between the jet and the vessel wall, slower moving and recirculating flow emerges. With increasing flow velocities, the formed vortices are shed downstream [19]. As these shedded vortices flow away from the stenosis, they break up into smaller and faster vortices very much like a Kolmogorov cascade. Examples of pulsatile flow through symmetric stenoses at 50%, 57% and 70% obstructions are illustrated in figure 2.15, where the obstruction is defined as $100 \cdot (D-d)/D$ [117]. It can be seen that for low flow velocities, a rather stationary vortex develops downstream of the stenosis. At higher flow velocities, an array of traveling vortices forms, rotating in opposite directions.

Numerous studies have correlated acoustic measurements with associated pathologies, see Ask et al. and references therein [19]. Common observations are that the sound intensity as well as the amount of higher frequencies generally increase with stenosis severity and that the recorded sound signal varies with the geometry of the obstruction. It has also been noted that the tube-wall vibration spectra can differ significantly from the turbulence spectra due to the tube's frequency dependent mobility. Further insight is limited, and more research is necessary [248].

Using bioacoustical techniques, stenotic vessels with occlusions as small as 25% have been detected [16]. Figure 2.16 indicates the onset of vascular murmurs as a function of Reynolds number. If peak systole produces a Reynolds number of 2000, then almost any degree of stenosis is capable of producing an audible murmur. On the other hand, if peak systole only reaches a Reynolds number of 500, a stenosis of less than 50% can not produce a murmur. It should however be noted that very severe obstructions (more than 95%) may not produce any sounds at all due to low blood flow [204].

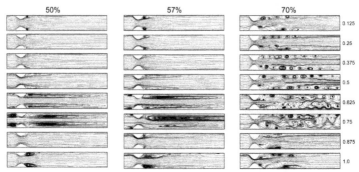

Fig. 2.15: Instantaneous streamline patterns at different time instances (indicated by numbers on the right-hand side) over systole and early diastole (top to bottom) and at increasing severity of the stenosis (50%, 57% and 70%). The image is the result from a simulation study using the finite volume method [117]. It should be noted that this is just an illustrative example. As mentioned in the main text, the onset of turbulence depends not only on the geometry of the stenosis, but also on the frequency of the pulsatile flow. Here the heart rate was 1 Hz, with flow velocities ranging from -0.04 to 0.26 m/s, see Jung et al. [117] for details. Image adopted from Jung et al. [117], with permission.

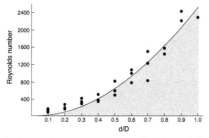

Fig. 2.16: The onset of vascular murmurs as a function of Reynolds number and percent stenosis measured in the aorta of a dog. The white area represents a flow condition capable of producing murmurs whereas flow conditions represented by the grey area will not produce murmurs. The curve is the least squares parabola best fit to the measured data points. Figure based on data and diagram from Sacks et al. [204].

2.6 Models of cardiac sound

The main motivation for model construction is to gain understanding about the physical world. A model is often realized by a set of equations that summarize available knowledge and set up rules for how this knowledge interacts. Modeling the cardiovascular system requires multi-variate, multi-scale, multi-organ integration of information, making it an extremely difficult task. The purpose of this section is not to delve into these details but rather to look at two simple models able to reproduce S1 and S2. Neither of the models is able to explain the genesis of the heart sounds. However, they do provide adequate representations of the PCG signal, and as such, the models can be used to simulate heart sounds. The models of S1 and S2 will be used to investigate robustness to noise and to define design parameters in chapter 4.

A different kind of model with a different area of application is the animal model. The purpose of these models is usually to perform provocations which are not ethically justifiable in humans. In this book, animal models are used for a more benevolent reason: the prevalence of certain heart diseases is very high in certain species, and the progression of the disease is often accelerated compared to humans. The dog models will be used in chapter 5.

2.6.1 Modeling the first heart sound

Models of S1 are somewhat ad hoc since the underlying mechanisms of the sound are not fully understood. Based on observations from thoracic surface recordings, Chen et al. [42] suggested a model consisting of two valvular components with constant frequency and one myocardial component with instantaneously increasing frequency. The basic idea is that harmonic oscillations associated with atrioventricular valve closure are dampened by the acoustic transmission to the thoracic surface. The valvular components $s_v(t)$ are modeled as a set of transient deterministic signals according to equation 2.3, where N is the number of components, A_i is the amplitude and φ_i is the frequency function of the ith sinusoid.

$$s_v(t) = \sum_{i=1}^{N} A_i(t) \sin(\varphi_i(t)) \qquad (2.3)$$

The myocardial component, associated with myocardial tension, is modeled with an amplitude modulated linear chirp according to equation 2.4. $A_m(t)$ is the amplitude modulating wave and $\varphi_m(t)$ is the frequency function. The frequency of the signal increases during myocardial contraction and levels out as the force plateau is reached [42]. Since the valves close after contraction, the valvular components and the myocardial component are separated by a time delay t_0 before attaining the final S1 model (equation 2.5). Figure 2.17 shows an example of the two valvular components, the myocardial component and the resulting synthesized S1 signal.

$$s_m(t) = A_m(t)sin(\varphi_m(t)) \qquad (2.4)$$

$$S_1(t) = s_m(t) + \begin{cases} 0 & 0 \leq t \leq t_0 \\ s_v(t - t_0) & t \geq t_0 \end{cases} \qquad (2.5)$$

For theoretical simulation of S1, Chen et al. [42] suggest the following functions ($N = 2$, $0 \leq t \leq 100$ ms, $t_0 = 10$ ms):

$$s_v(t) = e^{-60t} \sin\left(2\pi(50)t - \pi\right) + 0.5e^{-60t} \sin\left(2\pi(150)t - \pi\right)$$

35

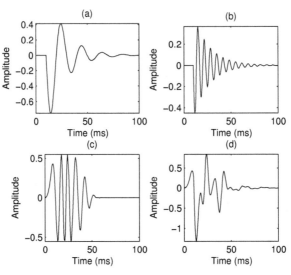

Fig. 2.17: Basic characteristics of the two valvular components, (a) and (b), and the myocardial component (c) of a simulated S1 signal (d).

$$A_m(t) = \begin{cases} 0.275(1.1 - 0.9\cos(83.4\pi t)) & 0 < t \le 12 \\ 0.55 & 12 < t \le 30 \\ 0.275(1 - \cos(34\pi t)) & 30 < t \le 60 \\ 0 & t > 60 \end{cases}$$

$$\varphi_m(t) = \begin{cases} 2\pi\left(60 - 40\cos(34\pi t)\right)t & 0 < t \le 30 \\ 2\pi\left(100\right)t - \frac{2\pi}{5} & 30 < t \le 60 \end{cases}$$

2.6.2   Modeling the second heart sound

Compared to S1, the underlying mechanisms associated with S2 are more widely accepted. The aortic component (A2) is produced during the closure of the aortic valve while the pulmonary component (P2) results from the closure of the pulmonary valve. Each component usually lasts for less than 80 ms. During expiration the two components come closer together (<15 ms) while during inspiration, A2 and P2 are separated by 30–80 ms [246]. The separation between the two components is mostly due to different durations of ventricular systole for the left and the right side of the heart, which is modulated by respiration (see section 2.5.1).

As indicated by Bartels et al. [22] and Longhini et al. [143], the resonance frequencies of A2 and P2 are proportional to the pulmonary artery pressure and the aortic pressure, respectively. This is reasonable since these pressures cause tension in the cardiac structures and the tension affects the frequency of the vibrations. With decreasing pressure in end systole and early diastole, it is thus expected that the instantaneous frequency will decay. According to this hypothesis, A2 and P2 should be composed of short duration frequency modulated transient signals [245], giving an S2 model consisting of two narrow-band chirp signals, see equation 2.6. $A(t)$ and $\varphi(t)$ are instantaneous amplitude and phase functions, and t_0 is the splitting interval between the onset of A2 and P2.

$$S_2(t) = A_A(t) \sin\left(\varphi_A(t)\right) + A_P(t - t_0) \sin\left(\varphi_P(t)\right) \quad (2.6)$$

For theoretical simulation of S2, Xu et al. [246] suggest the following parameter values ($0 \leq t \leq 60$ ms):

$$A_A(t) = 1.5 \left(1 - e^{\frac{-t}{8}}\right) e^{\frac{-t}{16}} \sin\left(\frac{-\pi t}{60}\right)$$

$$\varphi_A(t) = 2\pi \left(24.3t + 451.4\sqrt{t - 1}\right)$$

$$A_P(t) = \left(1 - e^{\frac{-t}{8}}\right) e^{\frac{-t}{16}} \sin\left(\frac{-\pi t}{60}\right)$$

$$\varphi_P(t) = 2\pi \left(21.8t + 356.3\sqrt{t - 1}\right)$$

The first and second terms of $A_A(t)$ and $A_P(t)$ control the attack and decay of the instantaneous amplitude, while the third term ensures a finite duration of 60 ms. Taking the derivative of the instantaneous phase, it is clear that the frequency component of the two components decay very rapidly over the first 10 ms after which the decay slowly levels out. Figure 2.18 shows an example of a synthesized S2 signal using a splitting interval of $t_0 = 30$ ms.

2.6.3 Animal models and veterinary applications

The cardiovascular system in companion animals is similar to that in humans. The methods and theories of this book are therefore applicable for veterinary use as well. Due to breeding, some canine breeds have very specific diseases. For example, if a severe murmur is found in a boxer dog, it is very likely that the murmur stems from AS. The same situation occurs in the Cavalier King Charles Spaniel (CKCS), but here the murmur is most certainly from a leaking mitral valve. The high prevalence of certain diseases, in combination with the striking cardiovascular similarity between the dog and the human, has turned dogs into excellent research models [23]. Regarding canine heart sounds and murmurs, it has been indicated that they show great similarity to their human counterparts [110]. Another major advantage with dog models is that the progression of heart diseases is accelerated compared to humans. For example, CKCS dogs often develop MI during a relatively short period of time. Monitoring the progression of a disease during its development from a physiologically insignificant state to a severe state is thus practically feasible.

In this book, the boxer breed was used as a model for AS. The prevalence of heart murmurs in the adult boxer population has been reported to be up to 80% [98],

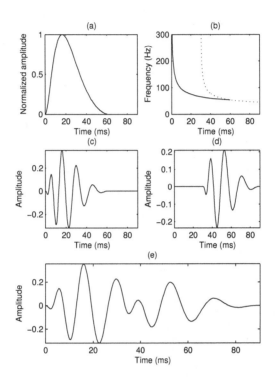

Fig. 2.18: Basic characteristics of the A2 (c) and P2 (d) components of a simulated S2 signal (e). Also illustrated are the normalized amplitude function (a) and the instantaneous frequency function of A2 (solid line) and P2 (dashed line) (b).

a high figure compared to other breeds of dogs. A proportion of the murmurs are caused by AS [172], but many of them are of uncertain origin. In contrast to humans, canine AS is not of degenerative origin, but a congenital disease affecting the aortic valves and/or the left ventricular outflow. There are also anatomical differences between the species. The human chest is flat while dogs have narrow deep chests. Therefore the heart is positioned closer to the thoracic wall in dogs and the heart sounds and murmurs are more easily distinguished. The differences in thoracic anatomy lead to different damping of the sound between the species. The amount of subcutaneous fatty tissue might also affect the damping of sound, a problem which is more prevalent in humans compared to dogs. However, the recording situation may be more difficult in dogs compared to adult humans due to practical reasons.

The Cavalier King Charles Spaniel will be used as a model for MI. Mitral valve disease is the most commonly acquired cardiac disease in adult dogs and it is the third most common cause of death in dogs under ten years of age [60]. Highest incidence of the disease is found in small to medium-size breeds, such as the Poodle, the Chihuahua, and the CKCS. Practically all CKCS have developed cardiac murmurs due to MI by the time they reach ten years of age. MI is commonly caused by myxomatous degeneration in the CKCS as well as in humans, and the compensatory mechanisms are also similar between the species [180]. The main differences in heart sounds and murmurs should thus be related to anatomical differences. Humphries et al. [110] suggest that the changed anatomy gives canine heart sounds a higher pitch, similar to what can be found in the human child.

3

Signal Processing Framework

*"Calling a science nonlinear is like calling zoology
the study of non-human animals."*
Stanislav Ulam (1909–1982)

The underlying assumption of many signal processing tools is that the signals are Gaussian, stationary and linear. The greater part of this chapter (sections 3.2–3.6) will introduce methods suitable for analyzing signals that do not fall into these categories. Two short examples are included in this introduction to illustrate the problems at hand.

Distinguishing signals with similar spectra: In many traditional linear methods it is assumed that the important signal characteristics are contained in the frequency power spectrum. From a stochastic process perspective, the first and second order statistics of the signal are represented by this power spectral information. However, there are many types of signals, both theoretical and experimental, for which a frequency domain representation is insufficient to distinguish two signals from each other. For example, signals generated by processes described by nonlinear differential or difference equations typically exhibit broadband spectral characteristics that are difficult to interpret and compare. Two signals with indistinguishable power spectra are presented in figure 3.1. The signal in subplot (a) is the logistic map while the signal in subplot (b) is its phase randomized correspondence. Even though they have the same frequency spectrum, the logistic map has structure in its phase portrait while the phase randomized signal does not (a phase portrait is basically the signal plotted against a time delayed version of itself). To distinguish between the two, or for that matter, to find the structure in the logistic map, it is obviously not enough to study the spectra of the two signals. This example was adopted from Povinelli et al. [190].

When putting together current analysis techniques and arranging them in a space spanned by nonlinearity and stochasticity, it becomes clear that this method space is quite sparsely populated, see figure 3.2. Periodic oscillations are found in the lower left corner (linear and deterministic), and these signals are usually analyzed with the power spectrum or by autocorrelation. This family of analysis tools will be presented in section 3.1. Linear dynamical rules, influenced by random external noise sources, are found in the lower right corner (linear and stochastic). Common

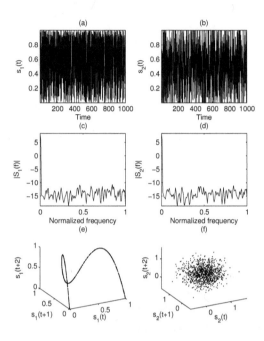

Fig. 3.1: The logistic map, $s(t+1) = c \cdot cos(t)[1 - s(t)]$, where c is a constant, is often used as a model in population studies. Here a logistic map with $c = 4$ and $s(0) = 0.1$ is presented in (a) and a phase randomized correspondence is shown in (b). Their respective frequency spectra, which are almost identical, are shown in (c) and (d). Finally, in (e) and (f) their corresponding phase portraits are shown.

approaches for dealing with these types of signals are linear parametric models such as the autoregressive (AR) model. Parametric signal processing techniques will be briefly mentioned in the end of section 3.1. Deterministic chaotic systems are found in the top left corner (nonlinear and deterministic). Such systems are controlled by strict mathematical rules, but even though the signals emanating from them might look abstract, an underlying order is inherently present. These signals are analyzed in a reconstructed state space and characterized by invariant measures such as the fractal dimension or the largest Lyapunov exponent. Analysis tools will be presented in section 3.4. When a system is driven away from the linear deterministic corner, higher order statistics are often more appropriate compared to spectral or state space representations [195]. Higher order statistics will be introduced in section 3.2. The linear parametric models in the lower right corner assume Gaussianity, but deviations from Gaussianity often contain pertinent information about the underlying system. Non-Gaussian statistics and various complexity measures are used to investigate the right border of the nonlinearity-stochasticity space, and such approaches will be introduced in section 3.3. The three corners containing

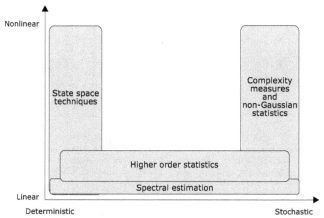

Fig. 3.2: Illustration of available types of analysis methods applicable to a variety of dynamical systems. Figure inspired by Quyen et al. [195] and Schreiber [207].

periodic oscillations, linear dynamics with external random noise and deterministic chaos rest upon a solid mathematical foundation where reliable and robust analysis tools are available. However, this doesn't mean that these areas are of particular interest, it only means that there are known methods to deal with them.

Changes in dynamics during the measurement period introduce nonstationarity in the signals. While these changes are often very interesting, most analysis tools ignore them altogether. This mismatch between the reality and the tools complicates the analysis. In the past, this problem was often dealt with by making sure that stationarity was established before the measurement phase begun. If nonstationary segments were detected in the data, these segments were either removed or the signal was split up into short quasi-stationary segments. A method able to investigate both linear and nonlinear nonstationary signals is described in section 3.6.

Time-varying frequency characteristics: A signal with multiple frequency components with changing frequencies is shown in figure 3.3. The signal consists of three components; a sinusoidal frequency modulation followed by a pure tone simultaneously with a chirp component. Using the Fourier transform to investigate the signal's frequency content, it can be seen that the signal contains a rather wide frequency peak. However, much more information can be obtained by investigating how the frequency content varies over time. As can be seen in the figure, all three signal components can successfully be detected using the joint time-frequency analysis tools that will be introduced in section 3.6.

The remainder of this chapter will deal with the two related topics of denoising and prediction (sections 3.7–3.8). A brief survey on classification (section 3.9), feature selection (section 3.10) and system evaluation (section 3.11) is also included.

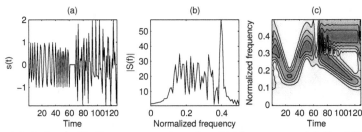

Fig. 3.3: A signal with three components, a sinusoidal frequency modulation followed by a pure tone simultaneous with a chirp component (a). The absolute value of the signal's Fourier transform reveals little of the three components (b). However, the combined time-frequency representation clearly exposes the individual constituents (c).

3.1 Linear correlations and the power spectrum

Irregular data sequences can be seen as stochastic processes, where the occurrence of a certain measurement at a certain time is regarded as a value drawn from a probability density function. The probability distribution is not known beforehand, but it may be estimated from the data, for example by a histogram. Descriptive measures of stochastic processes include the expected value and the variance. For a signal $s(t)$, $t = 1, 2, \ldots, N$, the expected value is defined according to equation 3.1 whereas the variance is estimated in equation 3.2. The standard deviation, σ, is defined as the square root of the variance.

$$\langle s \rangle = \frac{1}{N} \sum_{t=1}^{N} s(t) \tag{3.1}$$

$$\sigma^2 = \frac{1}{N-1} \sum_{t=1}^{N} (s(t) - \langle s \rangle)^2 \tag{3.2}$$

The time order of samples in $s(t)$ does not affect the mean or the variance, and to study time dependence, the autocorrelation function $c(\tau)$ is often used (equation 3.3). If $s(t)$ correlates with a time delayed version of itself, $s(t - \tau)$, the autocorrelation function will have a large value at $c(\tau)$. Similarly, a negative correlation gives a negative value of $c(\tau)$ while uncorrelated data gives $c(\tau) = 0$.

$$c(\tau) = \frac{1}{\sigma^2} \langle (s(t) - \langle s \rangle)(s(t - \tau) - \langle s \rangle) \rangle = \frac{\langle s(t)s(t - \tau) \rangle - \langle s \rangle^2}{\sigma^2} \tag{3.3}$$

If the signal is periodic, the autocorrelation function will be periodic as well. However, when studying oscillations and periodicity, the Fourier transform (equation 3.4) is often a preferable method. In time series analysis, the Fourier transform converts the time domain signal into a frequency domain signal.

$$S(f) = \frac{1}{\sqrt{N}} \sum_{t=1}^{N} s(t) e^{2\pi i \frac{tf}{N}} \tag{3.4}$$

The power spectrum (the Fourier transform of the autocorrelation function) is typically used to analyze and identify peaks which occur at the system's dominant frequencies and at their integer multiples (harmonics). For time-discrete signals, the power spectrum can be estimated by squaring the absolute value of $S(f)$, $P(f) = |S(f)|^2$. This estimate, called the periodogram, has a number of weaknesses; (i) the discrete Fourier transform has finite frequency resolution, which leads to leakage (broadened spectral peaks) and (ii), the presence of noise causes statistical fluctuations which are of the same order as $S(f)$ itself [140]. A number of spectral estimation methods have been developed to circumvent these problems. Averaging adjacent frequency bins in the periodogram is one approach (Blackman-Tukey's method), but, if there is enough data available, averaging over several periodograms is preferable (Welch's method) [140].

Assuming that $s(t)$ can be obtained by linear filtering of a zero mean white Gaussian noise sequence, $v(t)$, power spectrum estimations can be obtained by parametric modeling. The most general linear model within this setting is the autoregressive moving average model (ARMA), which is a composite model based on both the autoregressive (AR) and the moving average (MA) models (see equations 3.5–3.7).

$$s_{ARMA}(t) = -\sum_{u=1}^{N} \alpha_u s(t-u) + \sum_{u=0}^{M} \beta_u v(t-u) \tag{3.5}$$

$$s_{AR}(t) = -\sum_{u=1}^{N} \alpha_u s(t-u) + v(t) \tag{3.6}$$

$$s_{MA}(t) = \sum_{u=0}^{M} \beta_u v(t-u) \tag{3.7}$$

The MA model equation describes a convolution filter, where the new signal $s(t)$ is generated by an M-order filtering of the input signal $v(t)$. The name MA comes from the fact that the filter smooths $v(t)$ by averaging its last M values. This procedure is also called a finite impulse response (FIR) filter. The AR model, also called an infinite impulse response (IIR) filter, uses feedback to represent the system. The next sample in $s(t)$ is determined by the N previous samples in $s(t)$ plus an innovation sample determined by $v(t)$. Depending on the application, $v(t)$ could either be a controlled input or noise.

The ARMA model is most easily understood via the z-transform[1], equation 3.8. Since the convolution in equation 3.5 can be expressed as a multiplication in the z-domain, the ARMA model can be interpreted as in equation 3.9. The transfer function will diverge at poles due to the AR-term while vanishing at zeros due to the MA-term. The number of poles and zeros determines the degree of freedom of the system.

$$S(z) = \sum_{t=-\infty}^{\infty} s(t)z^{-t} \tag{3.8}$$

---

[1]The discrete Fourier transform is a special case of the z-transform where $z = e^{-i2\pi f}$ (the unit circle).

$$S(z) = A(z)S(z) + B(z)V(z) = \frac{B(z)}{1 - A(z)}V(z) \qquad (3.9)$$

Power spectral estimates derived from the three models are determined by the weights α_u and β_u, according to equations 3.10–3.12. The AR model is appropriate for modeling power spectra with sharp peaks while the MA model is able to represent deep valleys. The more general ARMA model can handle both sharp peaks and deep valleys. How to determine the coefficients and selecting the model order is out of the scope of this text, but details can be found in any book on digital signal processing, for example Ljung [140].

$$P_{ARMA}(f) = \sigma^2 \left| \frac{\beta_0 + \beta_1 e^{-i2\pi f} + \ldots + \beta_M e^{-i2\pi M f}}{1 + \alpha_1 e^{-i2\pi f} + \ldots + \alpha_N e^{-i2\pi N f}} \right|^2 = \sigma^2 \left| \frac{B(f)}{A(f)} \right|^2 \qquad (3.10)$$

$$P_{AR}(f) = \frac{\sigma^2}{|1 + \alpha_1 e^{-i2\pi f} + \ldots + \alpha_N e^{-i2\pi N f}|^2} = \frac{\sigma^2}{|A(f)|^2} \qquad (3.11)$$

$$P_{MA}(f) = \sigma^2 |\beta_0 + \beta_1 e^{-i2\pi f} + \ldots + \beta_M e^{-i2\pi M f}|^2 = \sigma^2 |B(f)|^2 \qquad (3.12)$$

ARMA coefficients, power spectra and autocorrelation coefficients essentially contain the same information. This means that linear models are sufficient only when the power spectrum contains enough information. Weaknesses in the power spectrum to discover underlying patterns in nonlinear data were exemplified in the introduction of this chapter. Another example is provided by a signal consisting of randomly spaced unit impulses of random sign. The power spectral density of such a signal is constant. By removing every other sample and multiply the remaining samples with $\sqrt{2}$, the same power spectrum is retained. By repeating this process over and over again, the power spectrum continues to remain the same while the signal becomes very different from the original signal. Clearly, information about phase and relative time delays is missing from the power spectrum.

3.2 Higher order statistics

In power spectral analysis, the signal is treated as a superposition of uncorrelated harmonic components. For this assumption to be valid, the signal has to be linear (superposition) and Gaussian (independent frequency components). The power spectrum derives from the autocorrelation function, which is a second order function (since the signal enters the equation twice). By generalizing the autocorrelation function into higher orders, higher order statistics are obtained. In contrast to second-order statistics, higher order statistics are based on averages over products of three or more samples of the signal, thus allowing nonlinear dependencies among multiple signal samples to be evaluated. Assuming zero mean signals with unit standard deviation and limiting the order to four, the order moments (m) and their corresponding cumulants (c) are defined as equations 3.13–3.17 [111].

$$
\begin{aligned}
m_s^1 &= c_s^1 = \langle s(t) \rangle = 0 & (3.13) \\
m_s^2(\tau) &= c_s^2(\tau) = \langle s(t)s(t+\tau) \rangle & (3.14) \\
m_s^3(\tau_1, \tau_2) &= c_s^3(\tau_1, \tau_2) = \langle s(t)s(t+\tau_1)s(t+\tau_2) \rangle & (3.15) \\
m_s^4(\tau_1, \tau_2, \tau_3) &= \langle s(t)s(t+\tau_1)s(t+\tau_2)s(t+\tau_3) \rangle & (3.16) \\
c_s^4(\tau_1, \tau_2, \tau_3) &= \langle s(t)s(t+\tau_1)s(t+\tau_2)s(t+\tau_3) \rangle - 3\left(\langle s(t)s(t+\tau) \rangle\right)^2 & (3.17)
\end{aligned}
$$

If the signal is Gaussian, it is fully described by its first and second order statistics, and higher orders are equal to zero. On the other hand, if the signal is non-Gaussian, the cumulants represent higher-order correlations. As such, they also provide a measure of distance from Gaussianity. Interesting special cases in equations 3.14–3.17 are $c_s^{(2)}(0)$, $c_s^{(3)}(0,0)$ and $c_s^{(4)}(0,0,0)$, which represent the variance, skewness and kurtosis of $s(t)$. Complete characterization of a stochastic process requires knowledge of all moments. Generally speaking, moments correspond to correlations and cumulants correspond to covariances. Even though both measures contain the same statistical information, cumulants are preferred in practice since [167]:

1. Cumulant spectra of order $n > 2$ are zero for Gaussian signals and their polyspectra provide a measure of the extent of non-Gaussianity.

2. The covariance function of white noise is an impulse function and its spectrum is flat. Similarly, cumulants of white noise are multidimensional impulse functions with multidimensionally flat polyspectra.

3. The cumulant of two independent random processes equals the sum of the cumulants of the individual random processes.

The Fourier transforms of the cumulants, called polyspectra, are defined according to equations 3.18–3.20. The Fourier transform of the second, third and fourth cumulants are called the power spectrum, the bispectrum and the trispectrum, respectively. An example of a bispectrum is shown in figure 3.4. The bispectrum quantifies the presence of quadratic phase coupling between any two frequency components in the signal. Two frequency components are said to be quadratically phase coupled when there exists a third frequency component whose frequency and phase are the sum of the frequencies and phases of the first two components. Basically, the power spectrum represents the product of two Fourier components with the same frequency, whereas the bispectrum represents the product of three Fourier components where one frequency equals the sum of the other two [89]. Interesting properties of the bispectrum, besides its ability to detect phase couplings, are that the bispectrum is zero for Gaussian signals and that it is constant for linear signals. These properties have, for example, been used as test statistics to rule out the hypothesis that a signal is Gaussian or linear [102]. Due to symmetries, only a small part of the bispectral space has to be analyzed [167], see figure 3.5.

$$
\begin{aligned}
C_s^{(2)}(f) &= FT[c_s^2(\tau)] & (3.18) \\
C_s^{(3)}(f_1, f_2) &= FT[c_s^3(\tau_1, \tau_2)] & (3.19) \\
C_s^{(4)}(f_1, f_2, f_3) &= FT[c_s^4(\tau_1, \tau_2, \tau_3)] & (3.20)
\end{aligned}
$$

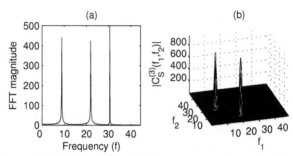

Fig. 3.4: **Example of phase coupling.** The frequency spectrum of a signal composed of three sinusoids with frequencies λ_1, λ_2 and $\lambda_3 = \lambda_1 + \lambda_2$ is shown in (a). The corresponding bispectrum is shown in (b). Since λ_3 is caused by phase coupling between λ_1 and λ_2, a peak will appear in the bispectrum at $f_1 = \lambda_1, f_2 = \lambda_2$ (another peak will also emerge at $f_1 = \lambda_2, f_2 = \lambda_1$).

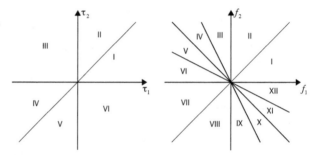

Fig. 3.5: **Symmetry regions of third order cumulants (left) and third order polyspectra (right).**

3.3 Waveform complexity analysis

There is an ongoing philosophical discussion about how complexity should be defined. An example of this quandary is that random noise has no structure at all, yet the term random perfectly describes the signal why it is easily described. Similarly, nonlinear equations such as Lorenz equations (see equation 3.32) are completely deterministic even though they might look obscure. Hence these types of signals are also simple. Thus, a system is simple when its dynamics are regular and described by a few variables. It is also simple when its dynamics are completely random. In between these extremes, where the system is a mixture of regularity and randomness, the complexity reaches a peak value [240]. From here on, this philosophical issue is left and complexity measures are merely considered as attempts to distinguish signals from each other.

In this section, a number of methods able to quantify complexity will be described.

The Hurst exponent $\mathbb{H}$, a measure of smoothness[2] in a signal, provides a link between several of these complexity estimates. More precisely, it can be shown that the Hurst exponent is related to the variance fractal dimension (VFD) of the $s(t)$ versus t curve by $VFD = 2 - \mathbb{H}$ [124] and to the slope of the curve's power spectrum by $\alpha = 2\mathbb{H} - 1$ [205].

3.3.1 Waveform fractal dimension

There are two principal approaches to estimate the fractal dimension of a time series, one that operates directly on the waveform and one that operates in a reconstructed state space [65]. Waveform fractal dimension estimates will be treated here while state space based estimates will be described in section 3.4.2. Note that the fractal dimension, measured in a reconstructed state space, is normally different from the waveform fractal dimension. The waveform is looked upon as a planar set in $\mathbb{R}^2$ where it is considered a geometric object. A line is a 1D object, a square is a 2D object and a typical time series has a dimension somewhere in between (since it is more complicated than a line but never covers the whole 2D space). Accordingly, the waveform fractal dimension is limited to the range $1 \leq D \leq 2$), where D is the dimension.

Even though there are many ways to estimate the fractal dimension of a waveform [65], only VFD is used here due to its robustness to noise [124]. VFD is calculated via the Hurst exponent according to equation 3.21. E is the Euclidean dimension which equals one for a 1D time series (thus reducing equation 3.21 to $VFD = 2 - \mathbb{H}$). In the VFD framework, $\mathbb{H}$ is determined via a power law relation between the variance of amplitude increments and their corresponding time increments according to equation 3.22, where $s(t)$, $t = 1, 2, \ldots, N$, is the signal and $t_{j,k}$ determines the j:th sample at scale k. By rearranging equation 3.22, an expression for H is obtained via equation 3.23, where C is a constant. If $\log var\{s(t_{j+1,k}) - s(t_{j,k})\}$ is plotted against $\log |t_{j+1,k} - t_{j,k}|$ for several different time increments k, $\mathbb{H}$ can be determined via the slope of a linear regression line, see figure 3.6(a).

$$VFD = E + 1 - \mathbb{H} \tag{3.21}$$
$$var\{s(t_{j+1,k}) - s(t_{j,k})\} \propto |t_{j+1,k} - t_{j,k}|^{2\mathbb{H}} \tag{3.22}$$
$$\log var\{s(t_{j+1,k}) - s(t_{j,k})\} = 2\mathbb{H} \log |t_{j+1,k} - t_{j,k}| + C \tag{3.23}$$

The choice of the time increment depends on the application. A unit time increment ($t_{j+1,k} - t_{j,k} = k$ for $k = 1, 2, 3, \ldots$) is preferred when separating a signal from noise while a dyadic time increment ($t_{j+1,k} - t_{j,k} = 2^{k-1}$ for $k = 1, 2, 3, \ldots$) is preferred for separating different components within the signal [124]. An illustration of the amplitude and time increments is shown in figure 3.6(b).

3.3.2 Spectral slope

If the power spectrum is inversely proportional to the frequency f according to some power law $1/f^{\alpha}$ [216], α can be interpreted as a complexity measure since

---

[2]The Hurst exponent reflects correlation between different scales of the signal

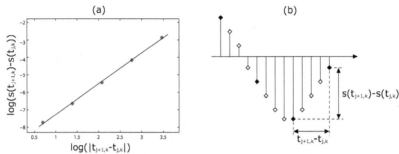

Fig. 3.6: A typical log-log plot (a), where the markers indicate the variance of amplitude increments at different scales. The dyadic time increment is illustrated in (b) for $t_{j+1,k} - t_{j,k}$ at scale $k = 3$ along with the corresponding amplitude increment, $s(t_{j+1,k}) - s(t_{j,k})$.

a large proportion of higher frequencies makes the signal look more complicated. In practice, the spectrum is plotted in a log-log scale, and α is estimated from the slope of the spectrum. For example, white noise is proportional to $1/f^0$, pink noise is proportional to $1/f^1$ and Brownian motion is proportional to $1/f^2$. Since $\alpha = 2\mathbb{H} - 1$, the spectral slope is related to VFD as $\alpha = 3 - 2 \cdot VFD$.

3.3.3 Entropy

Entropy is a generalization of variance to processes with non-Gaussian distributions [64]. As such, it can be used to describe system randomness and predictability, where greater entropy is associated with more randomness and less system order. As with the fractal dimension, entropy can be estimated either on the waveform or in a reconstructed state space, where the latter topic will be discussed in section 3.4.4.

There are a number of definitions available to estimate entropy. The Shannon entropy is defined in equation 3.24, where S is a discrete random variable with a set of possible values Υ and probability function $p(s(i)) = P\{S = s(i)\}, s(i) \in \Upsilon$. Basically, entropy describes how many binary (yes/no) questions that are required to find out the particular value of $s(i)$. The i:th value has an uncertainty $-log_2 p(s(i))$, and the sum provides the weighted average uncertainty. The log-function provides additivity such that uncertainties from different systems can be added together. $H(S)$ can range from 0, if there is only one possible value, to $log_2 N$, if all values of $s(t)$ are equally probable [74]. For experimental data, the probability density function has to be estimated, for example with a histogram.

$$H(S) = - \sum_{s(i) \in \Upsilon} p(s(i)) log_2 p(s(i)) \qquad (3.24)$$

Approximate entropy and sample entropy
Approximate entropy and sample entropy are two alternative measures of system

regularity. Given the time series $s(t), t = 1, \ldots, N$, a sequence of vectors $\boldsymbol{y}(t) = [s(t), \ldots, s(t+d-1)]$ is created. Each vector thus represents d consecutive samples, or patterns, in $s(t)$. The amount of vectors similar to $\boldsymbol{y}(i)$ is determined as $C_i^d(\varepsilon)$ according to equation 3.25, where Θ is the Heaviside function and ε is a tolerance level. The average amount of similar patterns of length d is accordingly given by $C^d(\varepsilon)$ in equation 3.26. This leads to the definition of sample entropy, equation 3.27, which measures the likelihood that patterns that are similar for d samples remain similar for $d+1$ samples [198]. Sample entropy was introduced as an unbiased successor to approximate entropy, which is similarly defined according to equations 3.28 and 3.29 [182]. In practice, these two complexity measures are nearly identical. More details about both of them will be revealed as the definitions are recapitulated in a reconstructed state space setting in section 3.4.4.

A short example showing how sample entropy values are calculated for a time series is illustrated in figure 3.7. A simulated time series $s(t)$ is used together with $d = 2$ and a tolerance level ε as symbolized by the dashed lines. Samples similar to $s(1)$ are symbolized by filled circles, samples similar to $s(2)$ are symbolized by filled squares and samples similar to $s(3)$ are symbolized by filled stars. Consider the two-pattern *filled circle - filled square* $(s(1)-s(2))$ and the three-pattern *filled circle - filled square - filled star* $(s(1) - s(2) - s(3))$. There are three occurrences of the two-pattern and two occurrences of the three-pattern, but since we do not count self-matches, they are reduced to two and one, respectively. These calculations are repeated for all two-pattern and three-pattern sequences, and the result enters equation 3.27 to determine the ratio between the total number of two-pattern sequences and the total number of three-pattern sequences. The sample entropy with $d = 2$ thus reflects the probability that sequences that match each other for two data points will also match for three points.

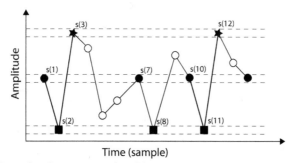

Fig. 3.7: Example of patterns analyzed by sample entropy. See the main text for details.

$$C_i^d(\varepsilon) = \frac{1}{N-d+1} \sum_{j=1}^{N-d+1} \Theta(\varepsilon - \|\boldsymbol{y}(i) - \boldsymbol{y}(j)\|) \qquad (3.25)$$

$$C^d(\varepsilon) = \frac{1}{N-d+1} \sum_{j=1}^{N-d+1} C_i^d(\varepsilon) \qquad (3.26)$$

$$H_{SE}(d,\varepsilon) = -ln\frac{C^{d+1}(\varepsilon)}{C^d(\varepsilon)} \qquad (3.27)$$

$$\Phi^d(\varepsilon) = \frac{1}{N-d+1} \sum_{j=1}^{N-d+1} lnC_i^d(\varepsilon) \qquad (3.28)$$

$$H_{AE}(d,\varepsilon) = \Phi^d(\varepsilon) - \Phi^{d+1}(\varepsilon) \qquad (3.29)$$

3.4 Reconstructed state space analysis

Dynamical systems theory is an important ingredient in nonlinear signal processing. A dynamical system is a system whose state changes with time. In continuous time, the system is described by differential equations and in discrete time by iterated maps. Since sampled data is used in this book, only iterated maps will be considered here.

The dynamics of a time discrete system is often described in state space, a conceptual space spanned by the dependent variables of the system. As time evolves, the system moves from state to state, tracing out a trajectory which provides a geometrical interpretation of the dynamics. If the trajectory is drawn to a particular set, this set is called an attractor. Examples of different attractors are given in figure 3.8. The transitions between the states can be described by vectors according to equation 3.30, where $\boldsymbol{x}(t)$ is the state of the system, t is the time index, ϕ is a mapping function such that $\phi^t : M \to M$ and M is the true state space.

$$\boldsymbol{x}(t+1) = \phi(\boldsymbol{x}(t)) \qquad (3.30)$$

The true state space (M) thus contains the true states $\boldsymbol{x}$, whose time evolution is described by the map ϕ, $\boldsymbol{x}(t) = \phi^t(\boldsymbol{x}(0))$. Now suppose that the only information available about this system is a scalar measure $s(t) = h(\boldsymbol{x}(t))$, where $h : M \to \mathbb{R}$ and $t = 1, 2, \ldots, N$. If $s(t)$ is a projection from M, it might be possible to undo this projection. That is, given a measured signal $s(t)$ in $\mathbb{R}$, is there a way to create a map from an unknown state $\boldsymbol{x}(t)$ in M to a corresponding point $\boldsymbol{y}(t)$ in a reconstructed state space in $\mathbb{R}^d$?

The problem of moving from observable quantities to theoretical notions was first solved by Packard et al. [176] who managed to reconstruct the state space based on a single scalar time series. A mathematical justification of this approach was later given by Takens [221], who proved that it is possible to reconstruct, from a scalar time series only, a new state space that is diffeomorphically equivalent to the original state space of the experimental system.

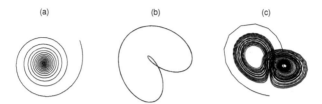

(a) (b) (c)

Fig. 3.8: Examples of a fixed point attractor (a), a limit cycle (b) and a strange attractor from a Lorenz system (c). A physical example of a fix point attractor is a pendulum, where all initial states will converge to a single point. Modifying this example so that the pendulum has a driving force, thus creating a simple oscillation, a periodic attractor is obtained. Chaotic systems like the Lorenz system have been used to describe weather, and give rise to strange attractors, where the trajectories never cross or touch each other.

There are essentially two methods available for state space reconstruction, delay coordinates and derivative coordinates. Derivative coordinates were used by Packard et al. [176] and consist of higher-order derivatives of the measured time series. This approach is motivated by the fact that any ordinary differential equation can be written as a set of coupled first-order equations. The system in equation 3.31 can easily be transformed into three first-order equations by setting $\psi = d\xi/dt$ and $\zeta = d\psi/dt$. In a Newtonian system, ξ, ψ and ζ would be the displacement, velocity and acceleration, respectively. The term $d^3\xi/dt^3$ is called the jerk [216]. The Greek variables should here be interpreted as the dependent variables spanning M, where one state is represented by the vector $\boldsymbol{x}(t) = [\xi(t), \psi(t), \zeta(t)]$.

$$\frac{d^3\xi}{dt^3} = f\left(\frac{d^2\xi}{dt^2}, \frac{d\xi}{dt}, \xi\right) \tag{3.31}$$

Even though the opposite is not necessarily true, some chaotic systems can be rewritten in *jerk form*. As an example, the Lorenz equations whose attractor was shown in figure 3.8 can be written in jerk form according to equations 3.32 and 3.33, where σ, r and b are model parameters. The bottom line is that a single variable ξ and its time derivatives can be used to describe the whole system. Unfortunately, since derivatives are susceptible to noise, derivative coordinates are not very useful for experimental data.

$$\begin{aligned}\frac{d\xi}{dt} &= \sigma(\psi - \xi) \\ \frac{d\psi}{dt} &= -\xi\zeta + r\xi - \psi \\ \frac{d\zeta}{dt} &= \xi\psi - b\zeta\end{aligned} \tag{3.32}$$

$$\frac{d^3\xi}{dt^3} = \left(\frac{1}{\xi} \frac{d\xi}{dt} - 1 - \sigma - b \right) \frac{d^2\xi}{dt^2}$$
$$\left[(1+\sigma) \frac{d\xi}{dt} - b(1 + \sigma + \xi^2) \right] \frac{d\xi}{dt} \qquad (3.33)$$
$$+ b\sigma(r - 1 - \xi^2)\xi$$

In rapidly sampled data, derivation can more or less be replaced by differentiation. An approximation of the derivatives in equation 3.31, expressed in delay coordinate terms, is given in equation 3.34.

$$\frac{d^3\xi}{dt^3} = f \left(\frac{\xi(t) - 2\xi(t-\tau) + \xi(t-2\tau)}{\tau^2}, \frac{\xi(t) - \xi(t-\tau)}{\tau}, \xi(t) \right) \qquad (3.34)$$

This is the starting point for Takens' delay embedding theorem, equation 3.35, where τ is a delay parameter, d is the embedding dimension and F is the map from the true state space to the reconstructed state space. A schematic illustration of Takens' delay embedding theorem is given in figure 3.9. This applies to almost every choice of $\phi(\boldsymbol{x}(t))$, $h(\boldsymbol{x}(t))$ and τ as long as d is sufficiently large (about twice the number of active degrees of freedom in the system), $\phi(\boldsymbol{x}(t))$ depends on at least some of the components of $x(t)$ and the remaining components of $\boldsymbol{x}(t)$ are coupled to $\boldsymbol{y}(t)$ via F [74]. Since the dynamics of the reconstructed state space contains the same topological information as the original state space, characterization and prediction based on the reconstructed state space is as valid as if it was made in the true state space. However, if the coupling between the observable and the system or between the dependent variables of the system is weak, the resolution available in an experimental setup will not be sufficient to rebuild the attractor [74]. Takens' theorem is only valid for deterministic and autonomous systems, but it may be extended to stochastically forced systems with slight modifications [218]. However, when dealing with recorded experimental signals, one should be aware that traditional linear techniques are probably more suitable.

$$F : M \quad \rightarrow \quad \mathbb{R}^d \qquad (3.35)$$
$$\boldsymbol{x}(t) \quad \rightarrow \quad \boldsymbol{y}(t) = F\left(\boldsymbol{x}(t)\right) = [s(t), s(t+\tau), \ldots, s(t+(d-1)\tau)] \qquad (3.36)$$

These ideas might sound far-fetched, but the same principles are used in the linear models introduced in section 3.1. Both the AR and the ARMA models use time lagged variables of $s(t)$. It seems like delay vectors are not just a representation of the state of a linear system – delay vectors can also be used to recover the geometrical structure of a nonlinear system. If the governing equations and the functional form of $s(t)$ are known, the Kalman filter is the optimal linear estimator of the state of a system [87]. However, when none or little information about the origin of $s(t)$ is known, state space reconstruction may help deducing clues about the underlying system.

Construction of the delay vector
The construction of $\boldsymbol{y}(t)$ suggests that the coordinates of a point in state space

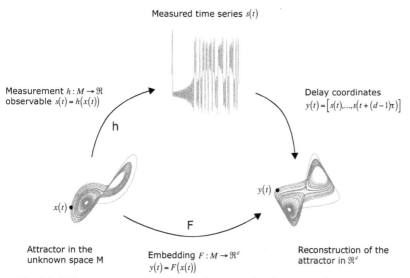

Fig. 3.9: Delay reconstruction of states from a scalar time series (example using the Lorenz system in equation 3.32). Redrawn from Parlitz [177].

correspond to the lagged amplitudes of $s(t)$. Regions in state space with similar coordinates will hence represent recurring patterns in the time series. It is possible though, that if the dimension of the state space is too low, states end up close to each other due to projection into a lower dimensional space instead of through the dynamics. An example is given in figure 3.10. The state $\boldsymbol{y}(t_1)$ is close to the state $\boldsymbol{y}(t_2)$ in the two dimensional space due to projection rather than dynamics. When the same attractor is represented in 3D, it is obvious that the two states are *false neighbors* in 2D. It is necessary to ensure that states in state space lie close to each other because of the dynamics and not due to projections. This process is referred to as attractor unfolding.

The selection of τ and d in equation 3.35 affects how accurately the embedding reconstructs the system's state space. However, for many practical applications the product $d\tau$ is more important than the individual parameters since the product represents the time span of the embedding vector $\boldsymbol{y}(t)$ [118]. This time window provides a snap-shot of the dynamics, representing one row in an embedding matrix according to equation 3.37.

$$
S = \begin{pmatrix} s(1) & s(1+\tau) & \cdots & s(1+(d-1)\tau) \\ s(2) & s(2+\tau) & \cdots & s(2+(d-1)\tau) \\ \vdots & \vdots & \ddots & \vdots \\ s(N-(d-1)\tau) & s(N-(d-1)\tau+1) & \cdots & s(N) \end{pmatrix} \tag{3.37}
$$

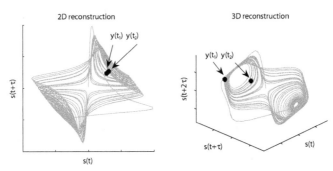

Fig. 3.10: Unfolding of the Lorenz attractor. In 2D there are false nearest neighbors in state space due to projection. In 3D, the former neighbors are far apart.

In this book, τ will be determined independent of d, after which d will be determined based on the selected lag value. How to choose d and τ is not obvious, and one should be aware that there are no bullet-proof methods available to determine the two embedding parameters. If the selection of τ and d are to be used in a particular application, it is often better to use some application dependent performance measure in the selection process.

The time delay
If τ is too short, each data point is too close together and the attractor tends to stretch out along the diagonal of the embedding space. On the other hand, taking τ too long leads to excessive folding of the attractor, see figure 3.11. The time delay τ should hence be long enough to make $s(t)$ and $s(t + \tau)$ independent and short enough so that the connection between $s(t)$ and $s(t + \tau)$ is maintained. Choosing τ as the first zero-crossing of the autocorrelation function (equation 3.3) is one approach, but this only establishes linear independence. A method able to detect both linear and nonlinear statistical dependencies is mutual information [70]. Mutual information quantifies the average information gained about one system, R, from the measurement of another, S, see equation 3.38. $H(R)$ in equation 3.39 gives the uncertainty of $r(t)$ in isolation, while $H(R|S)$ in equation 3.40 is the uncertainty of $r(t)$ given a measurement $s(t)$. The mutual information is thus a measurement of how much the knowledge about $s(t)$ reduces the uncertainty in $r(t)$. Since the logarithm is taken to the base 2, the unit of $I(R, S)$ is in bits.

$$I(S, R) = H(R) - H(R|S) \tag{3.38}$$

$$H(R) = -\sum_t P_R(r(t)) log_2 P_R(r(t)) \tag{3.39}$$

$$H(R|S) = -\sum_{t,u} P_{SR}(s(t), r(u)) log_2 \frac{P_{SR}(s(t), r(u))}{P_S(s(u))} \tag{3.40}$$

Usually, mutual information is measured between two different systems R and S. When investigating the mutual information within one system, but at different time

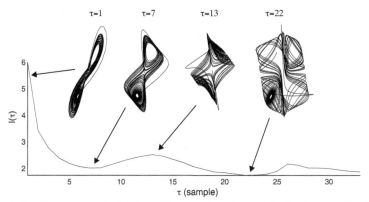

Fig. 3.11: The auto mutual information function along with the Lorenz attractor embedded for different time lags. The first local minimum in $I(\tau)$ facilitates a reconstruction where the attractor is properly unfolded.

instants, it is called auto mutual information (AMI). AMI thus quantifies the amount of information we possess about $s(t+\tau)$ based on knowledge from $s(t)$. When AMI is calculated as a function of τ, the AMI function $I(\tau)$ is obtained. AMI can be seen as a measure of the mean predictability of future points from past points in a time series and is often considered a nonlinear analog to the autocorrelation function [70]. The first local minimum of $I(\tau)$ represents a value of τ where $s(t+\tau)$ adds maximal information to the knowledge based on $s(t)$, and this value is often used to construct the delayed vector. There is no theoretical reason why the auto mutual information must have a minimum vale for a finite τ, but the results are eventually dominated by statistical fluctuations, why too large values of τ should not be considered as valid [216]. Possible reasons why there might not be a minimum in $I(\tau)$ could be poor signal to noise ratio, that the signal is undersampled or that too many degrees of freedom are present in the system.

Both the autocorrelation function and the auto mutual information function are useful when determining the time delay, but neither of them are consistently successful in identifying optimal time windows [153]. Essentially, none of them works for embedding dimensions greater than two since there are only two time instants that are compared. Further, the time lag does not have to be constant for each additional dimension. In fact, nothing but the complexity of determining adjustable time lags prevents delay vectors with variable τ. Such embedding procedures are out of the scope of this text, and a constant time lag will be used throughout this book.

The embedding dimension
The embedding dimension d should be chosen as twice the box counting dimension[3], but we have no idea how large this dimension is. One approach to estimate d is

---

[3] Actually, if the underlying system has n degrees of freedom, the embedding dimension required to recover these dynamics can be anywhere between n and $2n$, depending on the geometry [74].

the false nearest neighbors routine [118]. The basic idea is that if the attractor is not unfolded, two points can be near in state space due to projection rather than to actual closeness, see figure 3.10. To identify false neighbors, one compares the distance between neighboring states in dimension d, $\|\boldsymbol{y}^d(t) - \boldsymbol{y}^d_{NN}(t)\|$, with the distance between the same states in dimension $d+1$, $\|\boldsymbol{y}^{d+1}(t) - \boldsymbol{y}^{d+1}_{NN}(t)\|$, where $\|\cdot\|$ is some Euclidean distance measure. A false nearest neighbor is found if the ratio between the two distances, equation 3.41, is large. To determine the embedding dimension, the fraction of false neighbors is plotted for increasing dimension values, and a d-value is chosen where there are essentially no false neighbors left [216].

$$R(t, d) = \frac{\|\boldsymbol{y}^{d+1}(t) - \boldsymbol{y}^{d+1}_{NN}(t)\|}{\|\boldsymbol{y}^d(t) - \boldsymbol{y}^d_{NN}(t)\|} \tag{3.41}$$

This method is subjective since a threshold value has to be chosen to decide whether a neighbor is close or not. Cao [38] therefore suggested an extension to the nearest neighbor approach. By taking the mean value of $R(t, d)$ over all t, equation 3.42, a measure which is only dependent on τ and d (and not on the threshold) is obtained. Cao states that $E_1(d)$ stops changing when the number of nearest neighbors is constant, and this value of d is suitable for the embedding dimension. Note however that even noise reaches an asymptotic value for $E_1(d)$. An example of $E_1(d)$ plotted over a range of d-values for the Lorenz attractor is shown in figure 3.12. The knee-value where $E_1(d)$ stops changing is at $d = 3$, which coincides with the theoretical value for the Lorenz attractor.

$$E(d) = \frac{1}{N - d\tau} \sum_{t=1}^{N-d\tau} R(t, d) \tag{3.42}$$

$$E_1(d) = \frac{E(d+1)}{E(d)} \tag{3.43}$$

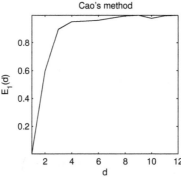

Fig. 3.12: Cao's method for determining the embedding dimension applied to the Lorenz system. A proper value where $E_1(d)$ does not change any more is $d = 3$, which coincides with the true value.

3.4.1   Characterizing reconstructed state spaces

It is always possible to use the method of delays to reconstruct a state space from any time series, but this does not mean that all time series provide meaningful structure in the embedded data. Because of the mapping between the true state space and the reconstructed state space, see figure 3.9, the precise values of $y(t)$ are not very interesting. However, the embedding $F(x(t))$ is smooth and invertible, so many important parameters about the system are preserved by the mapping. These parameters include invariant measures of the attractor such as dimensionality and the Lyapunov exponents (see the upcoming sections). Nonlinear deterministic analysis tools are rather different from their linear analogues, and a brief comparison between linear and nonlinear methods can be found in table 3.1.

Before applying these nonlinear analysis tools to an experimental time series, it should be tested whether it is likely that the data is nonlinear or not. A popular approach is the method of surrogate data, which can be summarized in the following steps [118]:

1. *Specify a null hypothesis.* Possible tests are that the experimental time series does not come from a distribution of independent random numbers or from a linear stochastic process with Gaussian inputs.

2. *Specify the level of significance.* A common choice is to use $p \leq 0.05$, meaning that the experimental time series should be different from the surrogate data in nineteen out of twenty cases.

3. *Create the surrogate data.* Surrogate data for the two tests in paragraph one could be created by a random permutation of the data or by randomizing the phase of the Fourier transform [208], respectively.

4. *Compute the test statistic.* The test statistic is a descriptive measure that is able to distinguish the nonlinear time series from the surrogate data. A simple nonlinear statistic is the higher order autocorrelation $\langle s(t)s^2(t+1) - s^2(t)s(t+1)\rangle$ which measures time asymmetry or the sample bicovariance (Hinich's test [102]). Other common choices are the dimension estimates that will be introduced in section 3.4.2.

These tests for signal nonlinearity are based on rigid assumptions such as the existence of a strange attractor. For real-world signals that are subject to noise and uncertainties, the rejection of the linearity null hypothesis have to be interpreted with due caution [148].

3.4.2   Dimension analysis

There are quite a few spaces and dimensions to keep track of when dealing with systems, attractors, embeddings and projections. There is a *configuration space* where the state equations live. It specifies the values of all potentially accessible physical degrees of freedom of the system. This space is often infinite dimensional. There is a *solution manifold* where the solution lives. This is the subset of the configuration space that the system actually populates as the dynamics unfolds.

Table 3.1: Comparison of linear and nonlinear signal processing techniques. The table is adapted from Abarbanel [1].

Processing task	Linear processing	Nonlinear processing
Finding the signal	Separate broadband noise from narrowband signal using spectral characteristics. Method: Matched filter in frequency domain.	Separate broadband signal from broadband noise using the deterministic nature of the signal. Method: Manifold decomposition or statistics on the attractor.
Finding the space	Use Fourier space methods to turn difference equations into algebraic forms. $s(t)$ is observed and $S(f) = \frac{1}{\sqrt{N}} \sum_{t=1}^{N} s(t) e^{2\pi i \frac{tf}{N}}$ is used.	Time lagged variables form coordinates for a reconstructed state space in d dimensions. $\boldsymbol{y}(t) = [s(t), s(t+\tau), \ldots, s(t+(d-1)\tau)]$ where d and τ are determined by false nearest neighbors and mutual information.
Classification	Use sharp spectral peaks and resonant frequencies of the system	Use Lyapunov exponents, fractal dimension measures, unstable fixed points, recurrence quantifications, statistical distributions of the attractor, etc.
Prediction	Find parameters α_k consistent with invariant classifiers - location of spectral peaks. $s(t+1) = \sum \alpha_k s(t-k)$	Find parameters a_i consistent with invariant classifier - Lyapunov exponents, fractal dimensions. $\boldsymbol{y}(t) \rightarrow \boldsymbol{y}(t+1)$ $\boldsymbol{y}(t+1) = F[\boldsymbol{y}(t), a_1, a_2, \ldots, a_p]$

Due to unexcited or correlated degrees of freedom, the solution manifold usually has a much smaller dimension compared to the configuration space. Lorenz equations provide one example, where the infinite physical degrees of freedom of a convecting fluid are reduced to three coupled differential equations. Thus, the manifold lives in a three-dimensional Euclidean space. Looking at the geometrical attractor of the Lorenz system (see for example figure 3.9, 3.10 or 3.11), it is also apparent that the attractor does not seem to fill the entire three-dimensional space. In fact, the attractor is very close to two-dimensional, or at least somewhere in between two and three dimensions (the Lorenz attractor has a *fractal dimension* of about 2.06). So far, we have been looking at the true system and the true attractor. As stated in the previous section, we observe this system via a (usually) one-dimensional measurement. This could be the velocity at one point in a fluid or the vibrations from a mechanical system. This *observable* is used to create a *reconstructed state space*, usually via the method of delays, in a space defined by the *embedding dimension*.

The fractal dimension of an attractor is invariant, even under different initial conditions. This explains why it is widely used for system characterization [65]. The fractal dimension cannot be calculated exactly from experimental data, but there are several estimation techniques, a few of which are:

1. box counting dimension.
2. information dimension.
3. correlation dimension.

Box counting dimension
The box counting dimension is based on how many d-dimensional hypercubes with side-length ε that are needed to cover the attractor. The required number, N, is a measure of how space-filling the attractor is. If the attractor has the hypervolume V, then the box counting dimension D_B can be determined from equation 3.44. Rewriting equation 3.44 into equation 3.45, a straight line with slope D_B is obtained. In practice, N is calculated for a range of ε, and D_B is estimated as the best fit line [4].

$$V = N\varepsilon^{D_B} \tag{3.44}$$

$$log(N) = D_B \log(\frac{1}{\varepsilon}) + log(V) \tag{3.45}$$

$$D_B = \lim_{\varepsilon \to 0} \frac{d \, log(N)}{d \, log\frac{1}{\varepsilon}} \tag{3.46}$$

Information dimension
The information dimension, D_I, is basically an extension of the box counting method. In both cases, the attractor is covered with elements of side length ε. However, where box counting just counts the number of hypercubes containing the attractor, the information dimension weights its count by measuring how much of the attractor that is contained within each hypercube [4]. The information dimension is defined according to equation 3.47 where $I(\varepsilon)$ is the Shannon entropy (equation 3.48). The probability function describes the probability of finding the attractor within the ith hypercube, so, if $P_i(\varepsilon) = 1/N$, the information dimension reduces to the box counting dimension.

$$D_I = \lim_{\varepsilon \to 0} \frac{I(\varepsilon)}{log\frac{1}{\varepsilon}} \tag{3.47}$$

$$I(\varepsilon) = - \sum_i P_i(\varepsilon) log P_i(\varepsilon) \tag{3.48}$$

Correlation dimension
The correlation dimension, D_2, is computationally more efficient and practically more feasible compared to the dimension estimates described above [4]. The correlation dimension is a measure of how the number of neighbors in the reconstructed state space varies with decreasing neighborhood sizes ε (equation 3.49). In theory, equation 3.49 should also contain a limit from $N \to \infty$, but in practice, N is limited by the sample size. This convey a lower limit on ε as well, since there will be a lack

of neighbors on short time scales. Further, finite resolution in the data inevitably causes errors at these fine time scales.

$$D_2 = \lim_{\varepsilon \to 0} \frac{d \, logC(\varepsilon)}{d \, log\varepsilon} \tag{3.49}$$

$C(\varepsilon)$ is the correlation sum as defined by equation 3.50. Θ is the Heaviside function, ε is the radius of a d-dimensional hypersphere centered on each point of the attractor $\boldsymbol{y}(t)$ for $t = 1, \dots, N$ and $\|\cdot\|$ is some distance measure. Basically, the sum determines the number of pairs of points in state space whose distance is smaller than ε.

$$C(\varepsilon) = \frac{2}{N(N-1)} \sum_{t=1}^{N} \sum_{u=t+1}^{N} \Theta \left(\varepsilon - \|\boldsymbol{y}(t) - \boldsymbol{y}(u)\| \right) \tag{3.50}$$

There are some practical aspects involved when determining the correlation sum from a time series. Firstly, the estimation in equation 3.50 is biased towards small dimensions because the data points entering the equation are not statistically independent [118]. This is due to *temporal correlations*, meaning that samples in the time series end up close together in the reconstructed state space, see figure 3.13. The neighbors that are not due to recurrent dynamics but rather from temporal correlations should be excluded from the correlation sum. This is easily taken care of by requiring a certain temporal distance between the states $\boldsymbol{y}(t)$ and $\boldsymbol{y}(u)$ in equation 3.50. A so called space-time separation plot has been introduced as guidance to determine a sufficient temporal distance, see Kantz and Schreiber [118] for details.

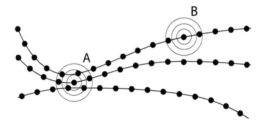

Fig. 3.13: **A 2D-projection of a reconstructed attractor. The circles represent hyperspheres with different radii ε around two different states A and B. State A have neighbors on dynamically independent trajectories while state B only have neighbors due to temporal correlation.**

Secondly, when calculating the actual dimension value (equation 3.49), it is customary to determine the correlation sum for several values of ε as well as for several values of d [118]. The results are plotted in a log-log plot according to figure 3.14, with $\frac{d \, logC(\varepsilon)}{d \, log\varepsilon}$ versus $log\varepsilon$. Three different scaling regions are commonly found in these plots. For large ε, the power law scaling turns invalid when the size of the attractor becomes small in comparison to the size of the hypersphere. This range of ε is called the *macroscopic regime*. Similarly, the *noise regime* explains the spurious results found for low values of ε. In the presence of noise, data points will be smeared out in the reconstructed state space, and for small ε this results in large errors. Even without the presence of noise, quantization errors and finite sampling will introduce errors in the correlation sum for small enough ε. In between these two regions, we find the *true scaling region*, and this is where we can calculate the correlation dimension. The larger the noise level, the smaller the plateau in the true scaling range will be. In the figure, it can be seen that $\frac{d\,logC(\varepsilon)}{d\,log\varepsilon}$ saturates at a value just above two in the true scaling region. This coincides with the true fractal dimension of the Lorenz system, which is about 2.06.

The problem of automatically choosing a scaling region is partially resolved by Takens' estimator, see equation 3.51. The sums are over all pairs of points closer than ε, so the equation is simply an average dimension for scales smaller than ε (with higher weights for the more nearby states). Takens' estimator offers better results compared to equation 3.49 for sparse, high-dimensional and noisy data [216]. The biggest issue with Takens' estimator is that the noise regime is included in the estimation [33], why it is better suited for distinguishing signals than for estimating their actual dimension.

$$T_2(\varepsilon) = \frac{\sum \Theta\left(\varepsilon - \|\boldsymbol{y}(t) - \boldsymbol{y}(u)\|\right)}{\sum log\left(\frac{\varepsilon}{\|\boldsymbol{y}(t)-\boldsymbol{y}(u)\|}\right)\Theta\left(\varepsilon - \|\boldsymbol{y}(t) - \boldsymbol{y}(u)\|\right)} \qquad (3.51)$$

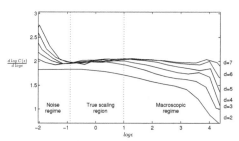

Fig. 3.14: Correlation dimension for the Lorenz attractor calculated for various embedding dimensions.

Thirdly, it requires a large amount of data to estimate the correlation dimension. There are no exact rules to determine how much data is enough since the necessary amount depends on the structure of the attractor. If the trajectories rarely visit some area of the state space, a very large number of points will be necessary to populate that region of the space. This applies to all kinds of fractal dimension estimates, not only the correlation dimension. Nonetheless, some rules of thumb have been suggested. If N is the number of relevant samples in the time series, the estimated correlation dimension should not exceed $2logN$ [59]. If the obtained estimate is larger than this limit, then the results are probably a reflection of noise and insufficient data rather than of a low dimensional hypothetical attractor [59]. Another suggestion for the necessary amount of data required to populate a state space is $N = 10^{2+0.4D_2}$ [216].

There are many more approaches available to estimate the dimension of an attractor, and most of them are described by Addison [4]. However, it is the correlation dimension which is used in practice. This is mainly because it is relatively easy to estimate, it provides a good measure of the complexity of the dynamics and it is computationally efficient [33]. Throughout this book, the correlation dimension will be used to estimate the fractal dimension of an attractor.

3.4.3 Lyapunov exponents

Maybe the most characteristic property of chaotic systems is their sensitive dependence on initial conditions. While many linear systems give rise to attractors with a slow rate of divergence, it is the exponential divergence that is characteristic of nonlinear chaotic systems. The most severe implication of this is that small causes do not necessarily have small effects. Lyapunov exponents quantify the average rate of convergence or divergence of nearby trajectories in a global sense. Positive exponents imply divergence, negative exponents imply convergence and zero exponent indicates a stable fix point (infinite exponents is a sign of noise).

The spectrum of Lyapunov exponents, λ_i, are defined in equation 3.52, where $J(p)$ is the Jacobian of the system as p moves around the trajectory. There is one Lyapunov exponent for each state space dimension, and each exponent describes the average rate of exponential change in an orthonormal direction, see figure 3.15.

$$\lambda_i = \lim_{n \to \infty} \frac{1}{n} ln \left(eig \prod_{p=0}^{n} J(p) \right) \tag{3.52}$$

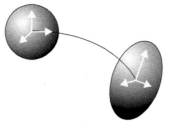

Fig. 3.15: Divergence and contraction of Lyapunov exponents in different directions.

Since the full Lyapunov spectrum is very difficult to estimate from experimental data, we will only look at the largest Lyapunov exponent [118]. A schematic drawing of two diverging trajectories is given in figure 3.16. Two nearby states with distance δ_0 evolve over a time period Δn and end up with a distance $\delta_{\Delta n}$. As this separation is exponential, it can be expressed as in equation 3.53, where λ is the largest Lyapunov exponent.

$$\delta_{\Delta n} = \delta_0 e^{\lambda \Delta n} \Rightarrow \lambda = \frac{1}{\Delta n} ln \left(\frac{\delta_{\Delta n}}{\delta_0} \right) \tag{3.53}$$

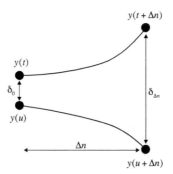

$$y(t + \Delta n)$$

$$y(t)$$

$$\delta_0$$

$$\delta_{\Delta n}$$

$$y(u)$$

$$\Delta n$$

$$y(u + \Delta n)$$

Fig. 3.16: Two exponentially diverging trajectories.

As in the Lyapunov spectrum calculation, the local Lyapunov exponents are estimated repeatedly along the trajectory and an average exponential change is taken as the final global largest Lyapunov exponent, equation 3.54. In words, the inner sum averages the distances from a reference state $\boldsymbol{y}(t)$ to its neighboring states $(\boldsymbol{y}(u) \in \Upsilon(\boldsymbol{y}(t)))$ Δn time steps ahead. The outer sum averages the local λ:s for each state in the trajectory.

$$\Lambda(\Delta n) = \frac{1}{N} \sum_{t=1}^{N} ln \left(\frac{1}{|\Upsilon(\boldsymbol{y}(t))|} \sum_{\boldsymbol{y}(u) \in \Upsilon(\boldsymbol{y}(t))} \|\boldsymbol{y}(t + \Delta n) - \boldsymbol{y}(u + \Delta n)\| \right) \qquad (3.54)$$

For robust determination of the largest Lyapunov exponent, $\Lambda(\Delta n)$ is calculated for a range of Δn, and if a linear scaling region is found, the slope of this region is set as the largest Lyapunov exponent [118].

3.4.4 Entropy

Entropy has been both mentioned and used in previous sections already, but so far without a proper introduction. There are many interpretations of entropy, a few of which are; the amount of energy in a system that is unable to do work, the energy dispersal at a specific temperature or the amount of information in a process [2]. Although there is a full family of entropies (the order-q Renyi entropies), only orders 1 (Shannon entropy) and 2 will be considered here. Accurate high-dimensional entropy estimates require tremendous amounts of data due to the high-dimensional probability distributions. One way to estimate the probability distributions is to partition the space into equally sized boxes (similar to the box counting approach for dimension estimation), thus constructing high dimensional histograms. This approach results in the Kolmogorov-Sinai entropy according to equation 3.55, where $p(k_1, \ldots, k_N)$ is the probability that the system is in hypercube k_1 at time δ, in cube k_2 at time 2δ and so on. ϵ is the content in each hypercube. The last equality in equation 3.55 derives from assumptions of stationarity and after application of the chain rule.

$$
\begin{aligned}
H_{KS} &= \lim_{\delta \to 0} \lim_{\epsilon \to 0} \lim_{N \to \infty} \frac{1}{\delta N} \sum_{k_1,\ldots,k_N} p(k_1,\ldots,k_N) log_2 p(k_1,\ldots,k_N) \\
&= \lim_{\delta \to 0} \lim_{\epsilon \to 0} \lim_{N \to \infty} \frac{1}{\delta N} H_N \\
&= \lim_{\delta \to 0} \lim_{\epsilon \to 0} \lim_{N \to \infty} H_{N+1} - H_N
\end{aligned}
\tag{3.55}
$$

Partitioning the state space into boxes introduces severe edge effects and poor scaling [118]. Instead, estimates of KS entropy, more or less based on the correlation sum, have been developed [58]. In these approaches, overlapping boxes (or spheres) are used, and the partition elements are not uniformly distributed in space but centered on each measured state. Two main courses of action have been chosen, one developed by Eckmann and Ruelle [58] which is based on Renyi entropy of order 1 and another developed by Grassberger and Procaccia [84] based on Renyi entropy of order 2. Let's start with some preliminary equations:

$$
C_i^d(\varepsilon) = \frac{1}{N-d+1} \sum_{j=1}^{N-d+1} \Theta(\varepsilon - \|\boldsymbol{y}(i) - \boldsymbol{y}(j)\|)
\tag{3.56}
$$

$$
C^d(\varepsilon) = \frac{1}{N-d+1} \sum_{j=1}^{N-d+1} C_i^d(\varepsilon)
\tag{3.57}
$$

$$
\Phi^d(\varepsilon) = \frac{1}{N-d+1} \sum_{j=1}^{N-d+1} ln C_i^d(\varepsilon)
\tag{3.58}
$$

Equation 3.56 is the probability that a state $\boldsymbol{y}(j)$ is close to the state $\boldsymbol{y}(i)$ in dimension d, and equation 3.57 is the average amount of neighbors to any state. Equation 3.58 is similar to equation 3.57, with the difference that $\Phi^d(\varepsilon)$ is the average of the natural *logarithm* of $C_i^d(\varepsilon)$.

Eckmann and Ruelle's entropy estimate is defined in equation 3.59. The expression is approximately $1/(N-d) \sum ln(C_i^d(\varepsilon)/C_i^{d+1}(\varepsilon))$, or in words, the average of the natural logarithm of the probability that states that are close to each other in dimension d are also close in dimension $d+1$. From a 1D perspective, this corresponds to the probability that patterns of length d continues to match when a new sample is added to the pattern (new length $= d + 1$).

$$
H_{ER} = \lim_{N \to \infty} \lim_{d \to \infty} \lim_{\varepsilon \to 0} \Phi^d(\varepsilon) - \Phi^{d+1}(\varepsilon)
\tag{3.59}
$$

Grassberger and Procaccia's entropy estimate is defined in equation 3.60. This expression is similar to the approximate value of equation 3.59, so the two estimates are closely related. However, the limits make both estimates cumbersome to calculate. In a real data set, the estimates can be reduced to statistic measures by limiting the amount of data (N). Further, the finite resolution of recorded signals and the presence of noise restrict both d and ε. In practice, the estimates should be stable over a range of d and ε values, otherwise the analysis is not reliable [118].

$$H_{GP} = \lim_{N \to \infty} \lim_{d \to \infty} \lim_{\varepsilon \to 0} -ln\frac{C^{d+1}(\varepsilon)}{C^d(\varepsilon)} \tag{3.60}$$

Approximate entropy and sample entropy

The entropy estimates in equations 3.59 and 3.60 (as well as the dimension estimates in section 3.4.2 and the Lyapunov exponent estimates in section 3.4.3) require careful statistical examination. For example, convergence of the correlation dimension does not necessarily imply chaos, but may also arise from an insufficient amount of data. Pincus [182] tried to somewhat relieve the constraints on the data when estimating entropy. This resulted in a measure, the *approximate entropy*, which is unable to certify chaos, but which is able to distinguish low-dimensional deterministic systems, chaotic systems, stochastic systems and mixed systems [182]. This rather strong claim is achieved by fixing the d and ε parameters in equation 3.59, resulting in a family of system equations, $H_{AE}(d, \varepsilon)$, equation 3.61. In practice, the amount of data is obviously limited, resulting in the family of statistics $H_{AE}(d, \varepsilon, N)$.

$$H_{AE}(d, \varepsilon) = \lim_{N \to \infty} \Phi^d(\varepsilon) - \Phi^{d+1}(\varepsilon) \tag{3.61}$$

Since the approximate entropy measure is biased, the slightly modified sample entropy measure was introduced by Richman and Moorman [198], see equation 3.62. The main differences are that sample entropy is based on equation 3.60 instead of equation 3.59, that self-matches are excluded and that $C^d(\varepsilon)$ and $C^{d+1}(\varepsilon)$ are defined to have the same length. The practical implications of these modifications are that sample entropy is less dependent on the time series length and that it shows better consistency over a broader range of possible ε, d and N values [198]. It should be noted that if the correlation sum defined in equation 3.50 is used, self-matches will automatically be excluded.

$$H_{SE}(d, \varepsilon) = \lim_{N \to \infty} -ln\frac{C^{d+1}(\varepsilon)}{C^d(\varepsilon)} \tag{3.62}$$

Changes in approximate entropy and sample entropy generally agree with changes in Eckmann and Ruelle's entropy estimate as well as Grassberger and Procaccia's entropy estimate [183]. Approximate entropy and sample entropy do, however, have four major advantages compared to the other entropy measures when used as a statistical measure to distinguish different systems [183]:

1. They are nearly unaffected by noise of magnitude below ε. For ε-values smaller than 0.1 times the standard deviation of the time series, one usually achieves poor probability distribution estimates, while for ε-values above 0.25 times the standard deviation, too much system information is lost. However, within this range, a suitable ε-value operates as an effective filter for noise cancellation.

2. They are robust to short bursts of both large and small artifacts since they have little effect on the probability distributions.

3. They give meaningful information with a reasonable number of data points. Sufficient estimates of the probability distributions require at least 10^d samples and preferably 30^d samples. This is similar to the data requirements for

calculating the correlation dimension, however, for distinguishing systems by approximate entropy and sample entropy, $d = 2$ is a common choice.

4. They are finite for both stochastic and deterministic processes. This is in contrast to the Kolmogorov-Sinai entropy which gives infinite results for random data. This difference is important since it allows approximate entropy and sample entropy to distinguish stochastic processes from each other.

3.4.5 Relations between invariants

Many of the dimension estimates are related through the so called Renyi dimensions. These measures define how different regions in state space should be given different weights. The Renyi dimension of order q is defined in equation 3.63, where $C_q(\varepsilon)$ is a generalization of the correlation sum in equation 3.50. Without delving into details, we just state that D_0 is related to the box counting dimension, D_1 is the information dimension and D_2 is the correlation dimension [118]. Similarly, as already stated, many of the entropy estimates are related by the Renyi entropies [118].

$$D_q = \lim_{\varepsilon \to 0} \frac{1}{q - 1} \frac{logC_q(\varepsilon)}{log\varepsilon} \qquad (3.63)$$

There are also relations between the different kinds of invariants. For example, positive Lyapunov exponents represent divergence of nearby trajectories. The fact that trajectories are diverging directly indicates that a lot of information is gained as time evolves. This link between Lyapunov exponents and entropy has been formalized in Pesin's identity, which states that the sum of positive Lyapunov exponents is a lower bound for H_{KS} [118]. Another example is the relation between Lyapunov exponents and fractal dimensions, where the Lyapunov dimension is defined in equation 3.64. D_L is equal to the information dimension for most systems [118].

$$D_L = j + \frac{\lambda_1 + \lambda_2 + \ldots + \lambda_j}{|\lambda_{j+1}|} \qquad (3.64)$$

3.5 Neural networks

Understanding the underlying dynamics of a time series by exploring its geometrical structure in a reconstructed state space is a possible route when such structures exist. When no typical structures or models can be found, neither from the linear methods in section 3.1 nor from the dynamical systems approach in section 3.4, it is possible to use a neural network to model the signal at hand [74]. A neural network (or some similar machine learning approach) can adaptively investigate a large space of possible models to find a working model which relates the input data to the output data. A drawback with neural networks is however that it is very difficult, if at all possible, to find out what the models really represent.

Neural networks are typically used for classification or pattern recognition where the task is to assign a number of inputs or features to one or more classes. This area of application will be treated further in section 3.9. In the time series setting, a number of old samples are presented to the network while the subsequent samples are used as target data. The task of the network is then to adapt itself to the dynamics of the system so that future data results as a function of previous data. An interesting observation is that temporal data is presented spatially as a time-lagged vector, just as in the previous sections. The network is thus trying to build a model of the reconstructed attractor.

A number of ingredients are needed to specify a neural network [74]:

- The interconnection architecture.
- Activation functions that relate the input of a node to its output.
- A cost function that evaluates the progress of learning.
- A training algorithm that updates the interconnections, or weights, of the network to minimize the cost function.

Figure 3.17 illustrates the most common network architecture which is based on three layers, an input layer, a hidden layer and an output layer. Each layer consists of a number of processing units, or nodes. The nodes in the input layer are passive (they do not modify the data), while nodes in the hidden layer and in the output layer are active (they modify the data according to the right-hand illustration in figure 3.17). Each active node can be seen as a correlation, where the weights α are adjusted to maximize the output when a certain pattern appears on the inputs. That is, the node calculates a weighted linear superposition of d inputs, $out = \sum_{u=1}^{d} \alpha_u s(t + u\tau)$. If the inputs are lagged values of the time series and the output is the prediction for the next value, each active node is equivalent to the $AR(d)$ model in equation 3.6. This also gives a hint on how to determine the weights. In the AR model, the coefficients are chosen to minimize the squared error [140], and the same approach can be utilized in the neural network setting. In defining the error $E = (out - target)^2$, learning is achieved by iteratively updating the weights in the direction that minimizes the error, by following the negative local gradient. This way, the new weights can be expressed as a function of the old weights according to equation 3.65, where η is the learning rate (or the step size taken in the direction of the negative gradient).

$$\alpha_u^{new} = \alpha_u^{old} - \eta \frac{dE}{d\alpha_u^{old}} = \alpha_u^{old} + 2\eta \underbrace{s(t + u\tau)}_{activation} \underbrace{(out - target)}_{error} \qquad (3.65)$$

When putting together several nodes into a network, it is possible to model more complicated functions. If each node represents a certain pattern in the input data, then subsequent layers look for patterns among the patterns. This is a very flexible structure since nonlinear interactions between the inputs are easily constructed [74].

Updating the weights in a multi-layer network is achieved by backpropagation, where each node is updated recursively using the chain rule of derivation. Even though more computations are necessary compared to the single node in the previous paragraph, the principle remains the same. Move in the direction of the negative gradient until you find the minimum of the cost function [18].

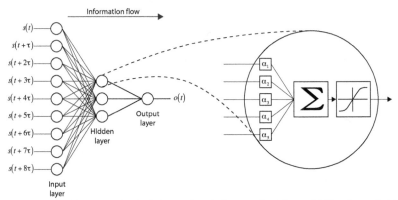

Fig. 3.17: Architecture of a feed-forward neural network with one hidden layer (left). A processing unit, or node, can be visualized as a flow diagram (right).

The sigmoid function in figure 3.17 is important for the network. It limits the output of the node by "squashing" the output from the weighted sum into a finite range. By doing so, the computing power of the network increases considerably [18]. Without the nonlinearity, an entire network with several hidden layers can be replaced with a single-layer network, thus reducing the network's modeling abilities to a simple linear AR-model [74]. Actually, any nonlinear "squashing function" can be used, but the sigmoid function is very convenient to use since its derivative can be calculated in an efficient manner.

In this section, we have only considered feed-forward neural networks, or more precisely multi-layer perceptrons. The network structure could be extended to not only send information forward, but to also include feedback paths. It is also possible to change the layout of the processing unit. One such possibility is the radial basis network. These matters are however out of the scope of this text.

3.6 Analysis of nonstationary signals

Stationarity requires that all parameters that are relevant to a system's dynamics are constant over time. Since the true system is unknown in most real applications, stationarity statements are often based on data from the system instead of from the system itself. Making stationarity statements based on data from the system instead of from the system itself is cumbersome since many stationary systems appear nonstationary when studied over a finite time period. How long a sufficient time duration of the measured signal is depends on the characteristics of the system under observation. As a first requirement, the duration of the signal should be much longer than the longest characteristic time scale relevant to the measurement situation.

Many signal analysis techniques presume stationarity. However, nothing prevents misuse of the algorithms by applying them to non-stationary data sets. Such abuse of the methodology does, however, cause results without physical meaning. For example, the Fourier transform has no time resolution and is thus unable to analyze nonstationary data. A solution to this problem is to use joint time-frequency analysis methods. Another example is that estimates of the correlation dimension suffer severely from nonstationary data sets. A simple drift increases the dimension (since all fractal structures are destroyed) while other nonstationarities or insufficient sampling rates yield spuriously low dimension estimates [118]. Tools to analyze both nonlinear and nonstationary data are not very well developed, but the recurrence plot in section 3.6.2 is one possibility.

Stationarity is a property which can never be positively established. However, the hypothesis of stationarity can be rejected by showing that the signal is nonstationary. Examples of tests include computations of the running variance or the running mean value of the signal [118]. Other important tests employ joint time-frequency representations to see if the frequency content of the signal changes over time [228].

3.6.1 Joint time-frequency representations

The *Shannon representation*, equation 3.66, of a signal is perhaps the most natural signal representation. The Dirac function $\delta(t)$ cuts out each observation of the signal $s(t)$, resulting in the waveform of the signal itself. In the Shannon representation, $\delta(t)$ is called an analyzing function, and when $\delta(t)$ is used to analyze the signal, perfect time resolution is obtained (see figure 3.18).

$$s(t) = \int_{-\infty}^{\infty} s(u)\delta(u-t)du \qquad (3.66)$$

A dual representation is the *Fourier representation*, equation 3.67, which was introduced in section 3.1. While the Shannon representation has perfect time localization and infinite frequency support, the Fourier representation has exactly the opposite qualities, i.e. perfect frequency localization and unlimited time support. The analyzing function in the Fourier transform is the exponential function. The time-frequency resolutions of the Shannon representation and the Fourier representation are illustrated in a combined time-frequency plane in figure 3.18.

$$S(f) = \int_{-\infty}^{\infty} s(u)e^{-i2\pi fu}du \qquad (3.67)$$

In order to capture nonstationary frequency components in a signal, the *instantaneous frequency* $\phi(t)$ needs to be defined. This is usually done via the analytic signal, $x_A(t)$. The continuous analytic signal is composed by the original signal and its Hilbert transform according to equation 3.68 where $s_H(t)$ is the Hilbert transform (equation 3.69).

$$s_A(t) = s(t) + i \cdot s_H(t) \qquad (3.68)$$

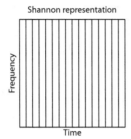
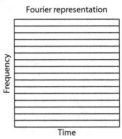

Fig. 3.18: Schematic illustration of the Shannon representation (perfect time localization) and the Fourier representation (perfect frequency localization) of a signal in the time-frequency plane.

$$s_H(t) = \frac{1}{\pi} \int_{-\infty}^{\infty} \frac{s(\tau)}{\tau - t} d\tau \qquad (3.69)$$

The Hilbert transform can be interpreted as a convolution between the signal and $-1/\pi t$, or as a rotation of the argument with $\pi/2$ for positive frequencies and $-\pi/2$ for negative frequencies. Similarly, the analytic signal can be obtained by removing the negative frequencies and multiplying the positive frequencies by two. The analytic signal possesses many interesting properties. For instance, the instantaneous envelope (equation 3.70), the instantaneous phase (equation 3.71) and the instantaneous frequency (equation 3.72) can easily be computed [83].

$$s_E(t) = |s_A(t)| = \sqrt{s^2(t) + s_H^2(t)} \qquad (3.70)$$

$$\phi(t) = arg\,(s_A(t)) = tan^{-1}\left(\frac{s_H(t)}{s(t)}\right) \qquad (3.71)$$

$$f(t) = \frac{d}{dt}\phi(t) \qquad (3.72)$$

Instantaneous frequency is a one-dimensional function of time, and as such it can only be defined for one value at each time instant. This implies that signals that contain more than one simultaneous frequency component cannot be analyzed properly using instantaneous frequency. Clearly, two dimensional signal representations with two dimensional analyzing functions are necessary.

The short time Fourier transform (STFT)

The short time Fourier transform, or the compressed spectral array as it is sometimes called, belongs to a group of *atomic joint time-frequency representations* (equation 3.73). The name comes from the two dimensional analyzing function $g(t, f)$, which is well-localized in both time and frequency, thus constituting an isolated island or atom in the time-frequency plane. As this analyzing function moves over the time-frequency plane, the signal's time-frequency content is gradually analyzed within the limits determined by the atom. The joint time-frequency transforms included in this chapter can all be interpreted as correlations between the signal and the analyzing function. In principle, the analyzing function represents one frequency, and the correlation procedure determines where in the signal this particular frequency exists. Next, the analyzing function is adjusted to represent a new frequency and the correlation procedure is repeated.

$$TFR(t, f : g) = \int_{-\infty}^{\infty} s(u)g(t, f)du \qquad (3.73)$$

The STFT is defined as a windowed Fourier transform (equation 3.74). The analyzing function $g(t, f)$ consists of an exponential function (just as in the Fourier transform) and a time localized window function $g_0(t)$, which is used to limit the time support. In practice, the Fourier transform is applied to short (possibly overlapping) segments of the signal, and the resulting spectra are stacked next to each other to obtain time dependency.

$$STFT(t, f : g) = \int_{-\infty}^{\infty} s(u) \underbrace{g_0^*(u - t)e^{-i2\pi fu}}_{g(t,f)} du \qquad (3.74)$$

The STFT, along with all other time-frequency decompositions, suffer from some uncertainty principle[4]. This basically means that it is not possible to know a signal's exact frequency content at a certain time instant. The frequency-resolution of the STFT is proportional to the effective bandwidth of the analysis window $g_0(t)$. Consequently, there is a trade-off between time and frequency resolutions: accurate time resolution requires a short window $g_0(t)$ while accurate frequency resolution requires a narrow-band filter, i.e. a wide window $g_0(t)$. If the time resolution is given by Δt_g and the frequency resolution is given by Δf_g, the uncertainty principle states that $\Delta t_g \cdot \Delta f_g \geq 1/(4\pi)$ [80]. The relation between time and frequency resolution is represented graphically in figure 3.19. Clearly, the area or the time-frequency atom is always the same whereas the height and width can be changed. Equality in the uncertainty equation is only achieved if g_0 is chosen as a Gaussian window function, see equation 3.75. The variance σ controls the width of the window and thus the shape of the time-frequency atom. This particular time-frequency representation is called the Gabor transform.

$$g_{gabor}(t) = \frac{1}{\sigma\sqrt{2\pi}} e^{-\frac{t^2}{2\sigma^2}} \qquad (3.75)$$

Wavelets
It is not possible to change the area of the time-frequency atom, but nothing prevents us from changing the width and height adaptively over the time-frequency plane, see figure 3.20. One idea is to analyze low frequencies with long time windows while analyzing high frequencies with short time windows. The Gabor transform uses a Gaussian window $g_0(t)$. By changing σ in the Gaussian function adaptively with frequency, a two dimensional analyzing function $g_0(t, f)$ is obtained. The width

---

[4]There are more than one uncertainty principle. The one mentioned here is valid for atomic time-frequency representations. Other uncertainty bounds apply for quadratic time-frequency representations [217].

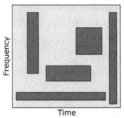

Fig. 3.19: The area of a time-frequency atom is always the same, however, it is possible to vary its width and height. The wavelet transform adjusts the shape of the atom depending on the frequencies that are currently under investigation.

of $g_0(t, f)$ is of short duration for high frequencies and of long duration for low frequencies. This particular time-frequency representation is called the Stockwell transform or the S-transform [220], and is defined in equation 3.76. The analyzing windows for three different regions of the time-frequency plane are illustrated in figure 3.21.

$$ST(t, f) = \int_{-\infty}^{\infty} s(u) \underbrace{\frac{|f|}{\sqrt{2\pi}} e^{-\frac{(u-t)^2 f^2}{2}}}_{g(t,f)} e^{-i2\pi f u} \, du \tag{3.76}$$

The S-transform is very similar to the wavelet-transform, equation 3.77. The main idea in wavelet analysis is that any signal can be decomposed into a series of dilatations or compressions of a mother wavelet, denoted $g_0(t, a)$. Just as previous analyzing functions, the mother wavelet is well-localized in time and frequency. However, since the wavelet function may contain more than one frequency, the link to local frequency is lost, and the term scale (a) is preferred instead of frequency. Each scale corresponds to a pseudo-frequency, which is the best possible fit of a purely periodic signal to the wavelet function, see figure 3.22. A number of standard wavelets are available (see figure 3.22 for a few examples), and as long as signal analysis is the main application, an appropriate choice is likely to be found in this library of known wavelets. However, in certain detection applications, where a certain waveform pattern is sought, custom made (matched) wavelets are useful. In this case, the mother wavelet should resemble the sought waveform in the signal.

$$WT(t, a) = \int_{-\infty}^{\infty} s(u) \underbrace{\frac{1}{\sqrt{a}} g_0(\frac{u - t}{a})}_{g(t,a)} \, du \tag{3.77}$$

The main difference between "classic" wavelets and the S-transform is that the S-transform uniquely combines frequency dependent resolution with absolutely referenced phase in each sample of the time-frequency plane. Absolutely referenced phase means that the phase information is always referenced to time $t = 0$. This is in contrast to a wavelet approach, where the phase of the wavelet transform is relative to the center (in time) of the analyzing wavelet. Further, the S-transform is sampled at the discrete Fourier transform frequencies, thus maintaining the notion

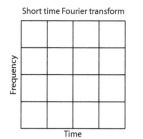
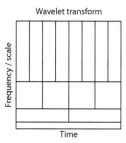

Fig. 3.20: Schematic illustration of the short time Fourier transform and the wavelet transform and their typical time-frequency patterns.

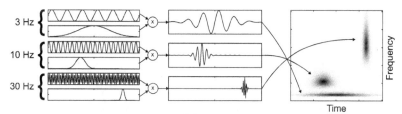

Fig. 3.21: The analyzing sinusoids $e^{-i2\pi ft}$ at three different frequencies together with their corresponding time-localized and frequency-dependent Gaussian windows $g_0(t, f)$ are illustrated to the left. Their products provide the analyzing function $g(t, f)$ at different time and frequency instants (middle plots). The area of the analyzing function (right plot) defines the region in the time-frequency plane where information is gathered about the signal.

of frequency [220]. An example comparing STFT, WT and ST is given in figure 3.23.

There are many other approaches available for joint time-frequency analysis. The methods just described belong to the linear nonparametric group. The quadratic nonparametric group, the parametric group etc., will not be treated in this book. An accessible review of these methods can be found in Hlawatsch et al [104].

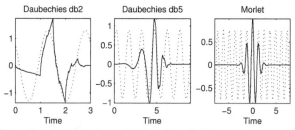

Fig. 3.22: Examples of standard wavelet functions (solid curves). Also included are sinusoids defined by the pseudo-frequency corresponding to the scale of the wavelets (dotted curves).

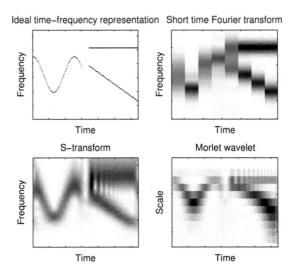

Fig. 3.23: Comparison of STFT, S-transform and wavelet transform based on the same example as in figure 3.3.

3.6.2 Nonlinear and nonstationary signal analysis

A joint time-frequency representation able to deal with both nonlinear and nonstationary data is the empirical mode decomposition [106]. Another approach is to combine wavelet analysis with the bispectrum, thus adding time resolution to the phase coupling information [230]. In this section, a third option will be described, namely the recurrence plot.

Recurrence plots

Nonstationarities reveal themselves as a tendency that points closely located in space are also close in time. Such observations can be analyzed by the recurrence plot, which was introduced to visualize high-dimensional state space geometries [57]. Normally, if a high-dimensional data set is to be visualized, the data is projected into two or three dimensions. Projecting the data into lower dimensional spaces do however fold the attractor, something that destroys its structure. Recurrence plots represent the recurrence of states of a system (i.e. how often a small region in state space is visited). A recurrence is a simple relation which simply states that a point in state space or a pattern in the time series repeats itself. Unlike other methods such as Fourier or wavelets, recurrence calculations do not require a transformation of the data [252]. Since no mathematical assumptions are made, recurrence plots are applicable to rather short time series from both linear and nonlinear systems.

A recurrence plot is derived from a distance matrix, which is a symmetric $N \times N$ matrix where a point (i, j) represents some distance between $\boldsymbol{y}(i)$ and $\boldsymbol{y}(j)$, $\|\boldsymbol{y}(i) - \boldsymbol{y}(j)\|$. Note that the distance matrix is invariant under isometries in state space such as translations, reflections and rotations. Thresholding the distance matrix at a certain cut-off value transforms it into a recurrence plot according to equation 3.78, where $i, j = 1, \ldots, N$, ε is a cut-off distance, $\| \cdot \|$ is some norm and $\Theta(\cdot)$ is the Heaviside function. An example of a recurrence plot is shown in figure 3.24. States that are close to each other in the reconstructed state space are represented by black dots in the recurrence plot.

$$RP(i,j) = \Theta\left(\varepsilon - \|\boldsymbol{y}(i) - \boldsymbol{y}(j)\|\right) \qquad (3.78)$$

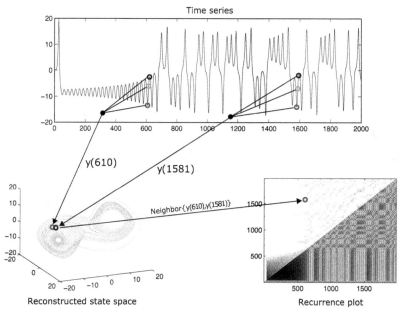

Fig. 3.24: Similar patterns in the time series end up close to each other in the reconstructed state space. This recurrence of neighbors is indicated by a black dot in the recurrence plot. The lower triangle in the recurrence plot has been replaced by a color coded distance matrix.

There are six parameters affecting the appearance of a recurrence plot; the embedding dimension d, the time delay τ, the range (or length) of the time series under investigation, the norm $\| \cdot \|$, the possibility to rescale the distance matrix and the cut-off distance ε [238]. Since recurrence plots can be very difficult to interpret [207], recurrence quantification analysis (RQA) has been introduced as a mean to quantify the plots. However, when the recurrence plot is summarized into a few scalar values, all time information is lost (and so is the information about nonstationarities).

Measures used for RQA are often based on diagonal structures, vertical structures and recurrence time statistics. Isolated recurrence points occur if states are rare, if they do not persist for any time or if they fluctuate heavily. Diagonal lines occur when a segment of the trajectory runs in parallel with another segment, i.e. when the trajectory visits the same region of the state space at different times. Vertical (horizontal) lines mark a time length in which a state does not change or changes very slowly. The most common RQA parameters are [72, 154, 237]:

- *Recurrence rate*: The percentage of recurrence points (black dots) in the recurrence matrix.

- *Determinism*: The percentage of the recurrence points that form diagonal lines. Diagonal lines are associated with deterministic patterns in the dynamics, hence determinism.

- *Laver*: The average length of the diagonal lines.

- *Lmax*: The length of the longest diagonal line. Lmax is inversely proportional to the largest Lyapunov exponent which describes how fast trajectories diverge in the reconstructed state space.

- *Entropy*: The Shannon entropy of the distribution of the diagonal line lengths. Measures the complexity of the signal.

- *Laminarity*: The percentage of recurrence points which form vertical lines.

- *Trapping time*: The average length of the vertical lines.

- *Vmax*: The length of the longest vertical line.

- *T1*: Recurrence time of the first kind, see below.

- *T2*: Recurrence time of the second kind, see below.

Nearest neighbors in the reconstructed state space can be divided into true recurrence points and sojourn points [72], see figure 3.25, where recurrence points of the second kind (T2) are the black states while the recurrence points of the first kind (T1) are all the states (black + white states). More formally, an arbitrary state, $\boldsymbol{y}(ref)$, is chosen somewhere on the trajectory whereupon all neighboring states within a hypersphere of radius ε are selected, see equation 3.79.

$$B_\varepsilon\left(\boldsymbol{y}(ref)\right) = \{\boldsymbol{y}(t) : \|\boldsymbol{y}(t) - \boldsymbol{y}(ref)\| \leq \varepsilon\} \forall t \qquad (3.79)$$

T1 is defined as all the points within the hypersphere (i.e. the entire set B_ε). Since the trajectory stays within the neighborhood for a while (thus generating a whole sequence of points), T1 doesn't really reflect the recurrence of states. Therefore, T2 is defined as the set of first states entering the neighborhood in each sequence (these points are commonly called true recurrence points). T2 is hence the set of points constituted by $B_\varepsilon(\boldsymbol{y}(ref))$ excluding the sojourn points, see figure 3.25. Both T1 and T2 are finally defined as averages over all possible reference states.

3.7 Noise reduction

Traditional linear filters are based on the assumption that the signal and the noise have distinguished spectra. In cases where the signal is broad-band and hence unseparable from the noise, other techniques might be more successful.

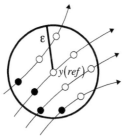

Fig. 3.25: Recurrence points of the second kind (solid circles) and the sojourn points (open circles) in $B_\varepsilon\left(y(ref)\right)$. Recurrence points of the first kind comprise all circles in the set.

3.7.1 Ensemble averaging

Welch's spectral estimation method, based on averaging several spectra, was introduced in section 3.1. The same principle is applicable to event-related signals in the time domain. If interesting signal patterns are triggered by a measurable event, then the signal can be divided into segments with appropriate length based on information from the the trigger. By simply averaging the derived segments, the maximum likelihood estimator for the pattern is obtained [217]. This assumes that the noise is additive, independent and Gaussian. It also assumes that the shape, duration and alignment of the signal pattern are constant. In the case when the noise is Laplacian, the median rather than the mean is optimal [217].

Assuming that each realization of the pattern $x_i(t)$ is additively composed of the true pattern $s(t)$ and some noise $v_i(t)$, then $x_i(t) = s(t - \theta_i) + v_i(t)$. By including a latency shift in the model (the random variable θ_i), some uncertainty is allowed regarding the timing between the trigger and the onset of the signal pattern. The estimated signal $\hat{s}(t)$, equation 3.80, can also be calculated recursively according to equation 3.81. The amount of new information that is recursively incorporated in the ensemble average can be controlled by replacing $1/M$ in equation 3.81 by a constant. Lower values of this constant implies that less new information is used while higher values only use the most recent segments in the estimation [87].

$$\hat{s}(t) = \frac{1}{M}\sum_{i=1}^{M} x_i(t) \tag{3.80}$$

$$\hat{s}_M(t) = \hat{t}_{M-1}(t)\frac{1}{M}\left(x_i(t) - \hat{s}_{M-1}(t)\right) \tag{3.81}$$

The latency shift θ_i can be determined with Woody's method [243]. It operates iteratively and start out by setting $\theta_i = 0$. This means that an initial estimate of $\hat{s}(t)$ is obtained by simply calculating the average across the ensemble of available segments. In the second step, each segment (or realization) of the signal pattern is pushed into place by employing a matched filter. If the noise is white and Gaussian, the best matched filter (in a maximum likelihood sense) is the time reversed $\hat{s}(t)$ estimate. Basically this means that the current segment $x_i(t)$ is cross-correlated with

$\hat{s}(t)$, and the time lag giving the highest correlation determines θ_i, see equation 3.82. Once every segment has been pushed into place, a new estimate of the signal pattern $\hat{s}(t)$ is determined. This process of translating and averaging is repeated until some stopping criteria is fulfilled. An example of ensemble averaging is presented in figure 4.5 on page 100.

$$\hat{\theta}_i = \underset{\theta_i}{\text{argmax}} \left(\sum_{\theta_i} x_i(t)\hat{s}(t - \theta_i) \right) \tag{3.82}$$

In cases with large latency shifts, it might be advantageous to use a predefined initial $\hat{s}(t)$ such as a triangular waveform [217]. A data driven alternative would be to use the most significant eigenvector of the ensemble matrix.

3.7.2 Wavelet denoising

Wavelet denoising is a powerful approach to noise reduction, especially when the amplitudes of the signal components are large compared to the noise amplitudes. The idea is to decompose the signal into a number of frequency bands. The resulting wavelet coefficients are then thresholded and transformed back into the time domain to obtain the denoised signal. Compared to linear filtering, it is more or less possible to preserve sudden changes in the signal while removing high frequency noise.

The definition of the continuous wavelet in equation 3.77 is highly redundant. By using dyadic sampling of the time $(t = k2^{-j})$ and scale $(a = 2^{-j})$ parameters, a more efficient signal representation is obtained. Instead of the two-dimensional time-scale representation, the full decomposed signal can then be fitted in a vector no longer than the signal itself. The discrete wavelet transform, with discretized time (k) and scaling (j) parameters, is defined in equation 3.83. W_{jk} is the kth wavelet coefficient at scale j, where $j = 1, \ldots, J$, $k = 1, \ldots, N/2^{J-j+1}$ and J is the number of scales that the signal is decomposed into.

$$W_{jk} = \int_{-\infty}^{\infty} s(t)g_{jk}(t)dt \tag{3.83}$$

Selecting a proper threshold is a crucial step in the denoising process. The so-called hard threshold function is defined in equation 3.84 and the soft threshold function is defined in equation 3.85. The hard threshold might create discontinuities in the results, something which is avoided by soft thresholding.

$$\tilde{W}_{jk} = \begin{cases} W_{jk} & |W_{jk}| \geq \eta \\ 0 & |W_{jk}| < \eta \end{cases} \tag{3.84}$$

$$\check{W}_{jk} = \begin{cases} \text{sign}(W_{jk})(|W_{jk}| - \eta) & |W_{jk}| \geq \eta \\ 0 & |W_{jk}| < \eta \end{cases} \tag{3.85}$$

Another threshold was developed by Donoho and Johnstone based on the the assumption of white noise [50], see equation 3.86. The factor $\sqrt{2 \ln N}$ is the expected maximum value of white noise with unit standard deviation and length N, and σ_v is the standard deviation of the measured noise. Various estimates of σ_v are available. If a global threshold is to be used for all scales, then σ_v is estimated as 1.483 times the median absolute value of the finest detail coefficients (this scale is assumed to contain as little as possible of the signal). The threshold can also be determined separately for each scale by using scale dependent estimates of σ_v, see figure 3.26. These thresholds correspond to an assumption of non-white noise and are derived by minimizing Stein's unbiased risk estimator. For nonlinear and possibly chaotic data, scale dependent thresholds should be used since uniform thresholding will undoubtedly remove important signal components [94].

$$\eta = \sigma_v \sqrt{2 \ln N} \tag{3.86}$$

Wavelet thresholding is simple and efficient but takes no advantage of the dependence between wavelet scales. Signals and noise behave differently in the wavelet domain, where sharp signal components evolve across scales while noise rapidly decays[5]. Multiplying adjacent scales will thus amplify edge structures and dilute noise. The multiscale products of W_{jk}, $P_{j_1k}^{j_2k}$, are defined as the product between adjacent scales j_1 to j_2. Thresholding is now based on the multiscale products instead of the wavelet coefficients, see equation 3.87. Note that for detection of transient signal components in noisy signals, the multiscale products themselves might be very useful.

$$\tilde{W}_{jk} = \begin{cases} W_{jk} & |P_{j_1k}^{j_2k}| \geq \eta \\ 0 & |P_{j_1k}^{j_2k}| < \eta \end{cases} \tag{3.87}$$

3.7.3 State space based denoising

If the data lies on a manifold, its geometrical structure can be used for denoising. This can either be done to smooth the manifold globally, or better, locally.

Global state space denoising
Singular spectrum analysis (SSA) is a method designed to extract information from short and noisy time series and thus provide insight into the dynamics of the underlying system that generated the series [63]. The technique is much related to state space reconstruction by the method of delays. In the method of delays, the reconstructed state vector is defined as $y(t) = [s(t), s(t+\tau), \ldots, s(t+(d-1)\tau)]$, while in SSA, an *initial* state vector is defined as $y(t) = [s(t), s(t+1), \ldots, s(t+m-1)]$. The SSA vector usually contains more samples compared to the method of delays vector. In the method of delays, the state vector spans a time window of length $(d-1)\tau$, and a window of similar length should be used in SSA. Since $\tau = 1$, a rather large m is needed to span a similar window.

From the initial state vectors, an embedding matrix with $\tau = 1$ is created, see equation 3.88 (the normalization ensures that $S^T S$ produces a covariance matrix). In the method of delays, the embedding matrix can be seen as a lag matrix multiplied by the identity matrix. Instead of multiplying with an identity matrix, any

---

[5]This behavior can be formalized with the concept of Lipschitz regularity [147].

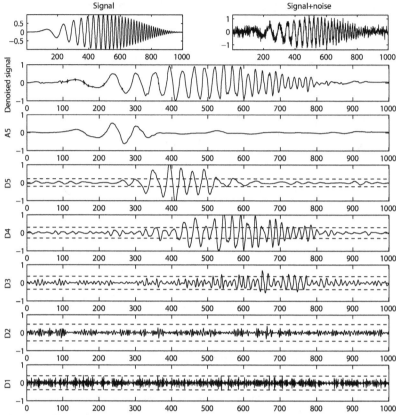

Fig. 3.26: Example of wavelet denoising with separately determined thresholds for each scale. The signal is decomposed into five scales using a Daubechies 4 wavelet, and Stein's unbiased risk estimator is used to calculate the standard deviation of the noise in each scale. The threshold is illustrated with lines in the subplots.

transformation can be applied. One idea is to multiply the lag matrix with a discrete Fourier transform, a low-pass filter and an inverse Fourier transform to get a smoother embedding matrix [74]. In SSA a similar but data dependent approach is used. By applying singular value decomposition to $\boldsymbol{S}$, the attractor is rotated in the embedding space so as to expose its largest face and reduce folding. In this way, the temporal structures that account for the maximum amount of autocovariance in the time series can be identified while additive uncorrelated noise can be suppressed.

$$\boldsymbol{S} = \frac{1}{\sqrt{N}} \begin{pmatrix} s(1) & s(2) & \dots & s(1 + (m-1)) \\ s(2) & s(3) & \dots & s(2 + (m-1)) \\ \vdots & \vdots & \ddots & \vdots \\ s(N - (m-1)) & s(N - (m-1) + 1) & \dots & s(N) \end{pmatrix} \tag{3.88}$$

In singular value decomposition, S is decomposed into $S = Q_1 D Q_2^T$, where the columns of Q_2 contain the eigenvectors of $S^T S$ and D is a diagonal matrix containing the square roots of the corresponding eigenvalues. If the signal is contaminated by additive uncorrelated noise, the largest eigenvalues will represent components containing signal plus noise while the smaller eigenvalues will represent components containing only noise. The idea is thus to first decompose the signal and then reconstruct it without the noise terms. This signal from noise separation is obtained by plotting the eigenvalue spectrum (called a singular spectrum), illustrated in figure 3.27. In such plots, an initial plateau with large eigenvalues contains most of the signal while the noise is characterized by much lower values. Hopefully these two plateaus are separated by a steep slope.

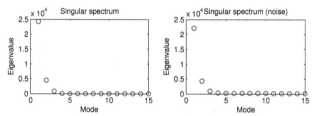

Fig. 3.27: **Singular spectra for the x-component of the Lorenz equations. In the right-hand figure, white Gaussian noise corresponding to an SNR of 10 dB has been added.**

To reconstruct the signal, the lag matrix is projected onto the eigenvectors (or principal components), $P = Q_2^T S^T$. Noise suppression is achieved by only using the columns in Q_2 corresponding to largest eigenvalues. The final reconstruction is achieved by summing up the reconstructed components in P (see figure 3.28 for an example). It has been argued that SSA provides better smoothing abilities compared to Fourier methods since SSA is data driven. Looking at the basis functions in figure 3.28, it becomes clear that the eigenvectors are very similar to Fourier modes, so perhaps SSA is somewhat overrated. After all, SSA is nothing but a linear root mean square fitting method, and Fourier analysis is optimal in the root mean square sense [35].

SSA has been suggested as an alternative embedding procedure to the method of delays. The steep slope in the singular spectrum indicates the embedding dimension, and the embedding matrix is constructed by using the corresponding number of reconstructed principal components as columns in the matrix. Quantitative interpretation of SSA results in terms of attractor dimensions has been heavily disputed [37]. One explanation is that the manifolds which contain attractors are not usually linear subspaces. Nonetheless, it has also been stated that these disputes originate from careless choices of m, and that the SSA approach outperforms the method of delays for noisy data [128]. Since SSA basically derives from the multiple signal classification (MUSIC) algorithm for spectral estimation, it is obvious that the reconstructed components are characterized by sharp spectral peaks. Consequently, embedding with SSA typically results in attractors with fixed points or limit cycles.

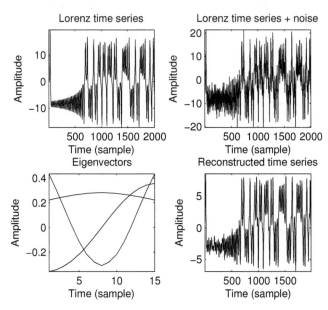

Fig. 3.28: **The x-component of the Lorenz equations are illustrated along with the same time series with 10 dB of additive white Gaussian noise. Three eigenvectors corresponding to the three largest eigenvectors are shown in the lower left-hand plot. The reconstructed time series was obtained by projecting the data onto the three eigenvectors and summing up the result.**

An example comparing time delay embedding and SSA embedding in the presence of noise is shown in figure 3.29.

SSA has also been suggested as a complexity measure. A trajectory with higher dimension causes a spreading of the singular spectrum. To quantify this spreading, the fractional spectral radius was developed [197], see equation 3.89, where λ_i is the i:th eigenvalue.

$$FSR(j) = \frac{\sum_{i=1}^{j} \lambda_i^2}{\sum_{i=1}^{m} \lambda_i^2} \qquad (3.89)$$

Local state space denoising
SSA analyzes the embedding matrix in a global sense, but since the manifold where the data lives is likely to be nonlinear, the linear principal components are not able to make the most of the structure in the data. However, since a manifold can be approximated locally by hyperplanes, other denoising approaches are conceivable.

An extremely simple nonlinear noise-reduction method based on local averaging in state space has been introduced by Schreiber [206]. The idea is to move each state vector $\boldsymbol{y}(ref)$ to the center of a local neighborhood in state space. The neighborhood can be defined as $B_\varepsilon\left(\boldsymbol{y}(ref)\right) = \{\boldsymbol{y}(t) : \|\boldsymbol{y}(t) - \boldsymbol{y}(ref)\| \leq \varepsilon\} \forall t$, so the current state

84

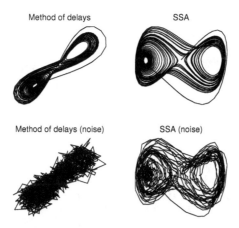

Method of delays   SSA

Method of delays (noise)   SSA (noise)

Fig. 3.29: Attractors reconstructed from the x-component in the Lorenz equations. The first column is reconstructed using the method of delays and the second column with SSA. The noisy embedding illustrates the effect of adding white Gaussian noise (SNR=10dB).

vector $\boldsymbol{y}(ref)$ is replaced by the mean value of $B_\varepsilon\left(\boldsymbol{y}(ref)\right)$ according to equation 3.90. The size of the neighborhood is determined by the threshold ε, and simulations shows that ε should be set to 2–3 times the noise amplitude [118]. Each of the state vectors is relocated using the original embedding matrix. Once all states have been moved, the whole procedure can be applied repeatedly. Convergence is typically achieved after 2–6 iterations [206].

$$\boldsymbol{y}^{new}(ref) = \frac{1}{\left|B_\varepsilon\left(\boldsymbol{y}(ref)\right)\right|} \sum_{\boldsymbol{y}(t)\in B_\varepsilon(\boldsymbol{y}(ref))} \boldsymbol{y}(t) \qquad (3.90)$$

A slightly more sophisticated technique is to apply principal component analysis to the neighborhood of states. Since the manifold can be approximated locally with a hyperplane, the idea is that the main principal components lie along the manifolds surface while the noise components are distributed in directions away from the manifold. By projecting the noisy states onto the space spanned by the main components, the noise is reduced. Examples of the two denoising methods are illustrated in figure 3.30. It should, however, be noted that these methods only perform well when there is a distinct structure in the reconstructed attractor.

3.8 Prediction

There are different sources of predictability in a time series. If the signal contains linear correlations in time, linear models such as AR (equation 3.6), MA (equation

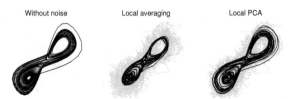

Fig. 3.30: Results from noise reduction using local averages and local principal component analysis (PCA). The Lorenz attractors were reconstructed from the x-component in the Lorenz equations with 10 dB white Gaussian noise added (gray).

3.7) or ARMA (equation 3.5) are suitable. As noted before, at first sight the classic AR model and the delay embedding might look similar since a prediction function is sought based on time-lagged vectors in both cases. However, a global AR model is designed to describe the data with a single hyperplane. If the data lies on a nonlinear manifold, the delay embedding can be used to describe, understand and exploit the structure in a better way.

The linear AR model can be expanded to allow nonlinear dependencies between previous outputs. Actually, a very general framework for predicting time series is given in Ljung [140]:

$$
\begin{aligned}
\hat{s}(t|\boldsymbol{\theta}) &= \sum_{k=1}^{N} \alpha_k g_k(\boldsymbol{\phi}) \\
\boldsymbol{\theta} &= [\alpha_1, \alpha_2, \ldots, \alpha_n]^T \\
g_k(\boldsymbol{\phi}) &= \kappa\left(\beta_k(\boldsymbol{\phi} - \gamma_k)\right) \\
\boldsymbol{\phi} &= [s(t-k), \ldots, s(t-1)]
\end{aligned}
\tag{3.91}
$$

All the g_k are formed from dilated and translated versions of a mother basis function κ. $\boldsymbol{\theta}$ is a vector of weights and $\boldsymbol{\phi}$ is a vector of known signal samples. α are the coordinates or weights, β are the scale or dilation parameters and γ are the location or translation parameters. A few examples of how this model framework can be used are [140]:

- *Autoregressive model*: set most of the parameters to unity.
- *Sigmoid Neural Network*: κ is a ridge construction such as the sigmoid function.
- *Radial basis networks*: κ is a radial construction such as the Gaussian bell.

If the underlying system is high-dimensional, has stochastic inputs or is non-stationary, neural networks are suitable for predicting nonlinear data. However, the hope that the network might learn the underlying structure in the signal comes at a cost. Neural networks are hard to interpret, and it is sometimes difficult to anticipate their behavior.

Returning to the reconstructed state space setting, it can be seen that $\boldsymbol{\phi}$ in equation 3.91 is very similar to a reconstructed state vector. By inserting a delay parameter

τ, or setting $\tau = 1$, ϕ becomes identical to $\boldsymbol{y}(t)$ in equation 3.35. One way to look at the model in equation 3.91 is thus as a global function describing the whole trajectory in a reconstructed state space. Usually, all parameters but the α:s are design parameters that either vary in a predetermined way or are fixed. Inserted into a cost function, equation 3.91 leads to linear equations when estimating the α:s, thus simplifying their determination [118].

That being said about global models, we will now focus on local methods to exploit the geometrical structure in the reconstructed state space. Local models can give excellent short-term prediction results and they are conceptually simple, but due to the dependence of nearest neighbor calculations they may be computationally demanding.

Similar trajectories in state space share the same waveform characteristics in time domain, and a way of predicting the future is thus to mimic the evolution of neighboring trajectories, see figure 3.31. If the data are sampled with high frequency, many of the discovered nearest neighbors are likely to be neighbors due to temporal correlations. A considerable improvement may thus be obtained by using nearest trajectories instead of nearest neighbors, see figure 3.31.

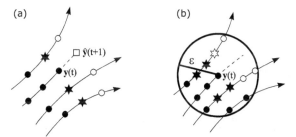

Fig. 3.31: Three trajectory segments and a (forward) predicted trajectory in a two-dimensional state space (a). The average change between the nearest neighboring trajectory points (black stars) and their successors (white circles) are used to predict the next point (white square). In (b), it can be seen that many of the nearest neighbors to $y(t)$, stars, are actually false due to temporal correlation. Using a nearest trajectory algorithm instead of a nearest neighbor algorithm may improve the prediction results.

There are two approaches to predict p steps ahead, either using *iterated* prediction or *direct* prediction. If the prediction is iterated, the algorithm predicts one step ahead p times (the predicted values will then be used together with the other states in the next iteration). In direct prediction, the evolutions of the nearest neighbors are modeled and the resulting function maps p steps into the future. It is empirically shown that iterated prediction is better on short term forecasts for a variety of nonlinear models. However, iterated predictions do not take the accumulated errors in the input vector into account, and these errors grow exponentially [156]. In *averaged* prediction, the average of the neighbors' successors (white circles) are chosen as the predicted value while in *integrated* prediction the next point is estimated as the current point plus the average change amongst the neighbors. If the trajectory that is to be predicted is an outlier, the mean of the nearest neighbors will always be misleading.

3.9 Classification

The design of a classification system is summarized in figure 3.32. The *sensor* and sensor data were described in chapter 2 and the *feature generation* has been described throughout this chapter in sections 3.1–3.6. The choice of features and the amount of features to use will be described in section 3.10. The selected features span a feature space, where each class is (preferably) clearly separated. The *classifier design* is about choosing and adapting a classifier able to draw boundaries between the classes. These boundaries are later used to assign unseen data to the most likely class. This could be done, for example, based on prior knowledge about the distribution of the various classes or on machine learning where a discriminative pattern is learned from the data. Different classifiers will be summarized in this section. Finally, when the classifier has been designed, *system evaluation* is the task to assess the performance of the system. This step is described in section 3.11.

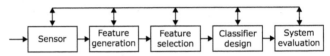

Fig. 3.32: The basic steps involved in the design of a classification system. Figure redrawn from Theodoridis and Koutroumbas [225].

Maximum likelihood classification
Maximum likelihood classification uses the probability density function for each class, and unseen data is simply assigned to the most likely class. A problem with the maximum likelihood classifier is that it can not handle multidimensional feature sets without estimating multidimensional probability density functions, and this requires a huge amount of data. An example of the probability density functions that a maximum likelihood classifier operates upon is illustrated in the right-hand side of figure 3.33.

Linear discriminant analysis
Linear discriminant analysis (LDA) is a transform-based method which attempts to minimize the ratio of within-class variance to the between-class variance. This results in a linear projection of the data onto the line that gives the maximum separation between the classes. Since the transformation reduces the feature space to one dimension, maximum likelihood classification can be used for the final decision.

k Nearest Neighbor classification
The k Nearest Neighbor (kNN) classification procedure is both simple and intuitive. Basically, unseen data is classified based on the behavior of its neighbors in the feature space. A distance measure is defined and the distance from the unseen observa-

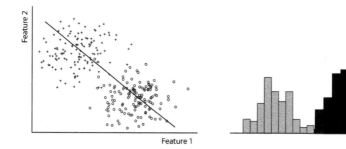

Fig. 3.33: Example with two features and two classes. The black line in the left-hand figure indicates the optimal projection vector obtained with LDA. The distribution of points after being projected onto the line is illustrated in the right-hand figure.

tion to all other observations is calculated. The k nearest neighbors are determined, and the unseen observation is assigned to the class that most of its neighbors belong to. A problem with kNN is that the computational complexity associated with nearest neighbor searching is rather high, especially for high-dimensional feature spaces. An example of kNN classification is illustrated in figure 3.34.

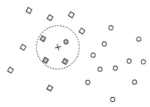

Fig. 3.34: Example with two features and two classes (boxes and circles). The unclassified observation ($\times$) is assigned to the box-class using kNN with $k = 4$ since a majority of the four neighbors are boxes.

Neural networks
Neural networks were introduced for system modeling in section 3.5 and for prediction in section 3.8. The most typical environment for neural networks is however in the pattern recognition domain. A collection of features are presented to the network, and the task is to adapt the weights so that the input features are nonlinearly mapped to two or more target classes.

3.10 Feature selection

Too many features often result in classifiers with low generality, and there are many potential benefits in reducing the number of features; facilitating data visualization, reducing the measurement and storage requirements, reducing training and utilization times and defying the curse of dimensionality [88].

3.10.1   Feature ranking

Scalar feature selection means that each feature is treated individually. A scoring function is defined, and its outcome indicates the predictive power of the feature. This way, all features can be ranked in decreasing order and the best ones are selected for the classification task. The scoring function could, for example, be the distance from the feature to the center of the distribution of the class it is supposed to belong to. Selecting the individually most relevant features is usually suboptimal for building a predictor, particularly if the selected features are correlated and thus contain redundant information [225].

3.10.2   Feature subset selection

A problem with scalar feature selection is that is does not account for combinations of features that together have great predictive power. An optimal selection requires an exhaustive search over all features, but this is practically infeasible. Instead suboptimal search algorithms are employed, many of which uses greedy hill climbing (hill climbing is a search algorithm where the current path is extended with a successor node which is closer to the solution than the end of the current path). A possible subset of features is then evaluated, and other features are successively added or removed from this set to see if an improvement can be achieved [88]. A simple way to do this is to start with one feature (the one with highest ranking according to scalar feature selection), say f_1. Expand the set to contain two features by forming all possible pairs, say $\{f_1, f_2\}$, $\{f_1, f_3\}$, $\{f_1, f_4\}$. The pair that maximizes some class separability criterion is selected as the new feature subset. More features are then progressively added into larger and larger subsets until the desired number of features is reached. This method is often used when the size of the final subset is supposed to be small compared to the total amount of features. If the final subset is supposed to be large, then all features could be included in a preliminary subset which is progressively reduced. These methods are called *sequential forward selection* and *sequential backward selection*, respectively. A common drawback for both of these is that once a feature is included there is no way of getting rid of it (and vice versa in backward selection). Pudil's sequential floating forward selection is a workaround to this problem, allowing features to be both included and excluded several times [192]. A flow chart describing the algorithm is presented in figure 3.35.

3.11   System evaluation

Evaluation and algorithm design can be done either on simulated data or on real data. Simulated data provides a controlled environment where everything is known while real data needs some kind of expert method or opinion to use as a reference.

Using simulated data, different algorithms can be evaluated in a quantitative and reproducible manner. Since the true signal is known, it is possible to add noise and evaluate the robustness of the algorithm or classifier. Depending on the data and the

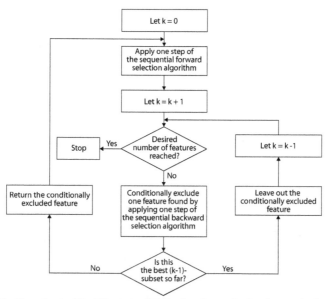

Fig. 3.35: Flow chart of Pudil's sequential floating forward selection method, where k is the current number of features in the subset. Figure based on a drawing by Pudil et al. [192].

output of the developed algorithm, different performance measures are of interest. For a change detector, mean time to detection, mean time between false alarms and average run length are useful parameters [87]. In the corresponding off-line application of signal segmentation, detection accuracy might be more revealing. For noise reduction algorithms, the mean square error between the noise-free signal and the denoised signal is a common criterion for minimization and the same criterion is useful for evaluating prediction algorithms. Obviously, the criteria for algorithm evaluation is highly dependent on the application at hand. The remainder of this section will deal with evaluating classification systems, especially for the case where representative data is hard to simulate.

3.11.1 Estimating classifier accuracy

In supervised learning, overfitting is likely to occur in cases where learning was performed for too long, where training examples are rare and/or where too many features are used in the feature vector. This basically means that many different solutions are consistent with the training examples, but disagree on unseen data. Hence, when presenting new examples to the developed classifier, the predictions will not be reliable. In order to avoid overfitting, it is necessary to use cross-validation to verify the results. There are three basic schemes for estimating the classification error probability [225]:

Resubstitution method: The same data set is used for training as well as for testing. Obviously this leads to a very optimistic estimate of the error probability. In order to get an accurate estimate, the number of test cases as well as the ratio between the number of test cases and the number of features should be large.

Holdout method: The data set is split into a training set and a test set. This approach requires a lot of data since only a subset of data is used in each step.

Leave-one-out method: All data but one case are used as training data, and data from the excluded case are used for validation. This procedure, in which a different case is excluded each time, is iterated for all cases. This means that basically all data are used for training and, at the same time, independence is maintained between the training set and the test set. The major drawback is the increased computational complexity.

Evaluating binary classifiers

To measure the performance of a binary classifier, the two concepts sensitivity and specificity are often used. If the system tries to classify persons to see if they have a certain disease, there are four possible outcomes. Persons with the disease can be classified to have the disease (true positives) or they can be classified not to have the disease (false negative). Persons who do not have the disease can be classified to either have the disease (false positive) or not (true negative). Thus, the number of true positives (TP), true negatives (TN), false positives (FP) and false negatives (FN) covers the whole set. Sensitivity, specificity, positive predictive value (PPV) and negative predictive value (NPV) are defined in equations 3.92–3.95. In words, these equations state that if the patient's disease status is known, then sensitivity means that "I know my patient has the disease. What is the chance that the test will show that my patient has it?". Specificity means that "I know my patient doesn't have the disease. What is the chance that the test will show that my patient doesn't have it?". If, on the other hand, the test result is known but the patient's disease status is not, then PPV means that "I just got a positive test result back on my patient. What is the chance that my patient actually has the disease?". Similarly, NPV means that "I just got a negative test result back on my patient. What is the chance that my patient actually doesn't have the disease?".

$$\text{Sensitivity} = \frac{TP}{TP+FN} \tag{3.92}$$

$$\text{Specificity} = \frac{TN}{FP+TN} \tag{3.93}$$

$$PPV = \frac{TP}{TP+FP} \tag{3.94}$$

$$NPV = \frac{TN}{TN+FN} \tag{3.95}$$

The outcome from a binary classifier in terms of TP, TN, FP and FN depends on the threshold which is used to separate the two probability distributions. A graphical representation illustrating how different thresholds affect the sensitivity and the specificity of the classifier is the *receiver operating characteristics* (ROC) curve, see figure 3.36. A successful classifier will result in an ROC curve tending towards the upper-left corner, while pure guessing results in a straight line at a 45° diagonal. The area under the ROC curve (AUC) is often used as a summary statistic since it relates to the Mann-Whitney U-test.

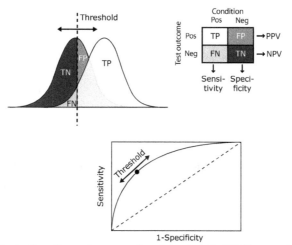

Fig. 3.36: Illustration of a receiver operating characteristic (ROC) curve. By altering the threshold, the amount of true positives (TP), true negatives (TN), false positives (FP) and false negatives (FN) also change. The subsequent changes on sensitivity and specificity are graphically illustrated in the ROC curve.

4

Heart Sound Localization and Segmentation

"Nothing is particularly hard if you divide it into small jobs."

Henry Ford (1863–1947)

Heart sound localization refers to the task of finding the normal heart sounds, but without distinguishing the two from each other. The main applications of localization are as a pre-processing step applied before heart sound cancellation (chapter 6) or before heart sound segmentation. *Heart sound segmentation* partitions the PCG signal into cardiac cycles and further into S1, systole, S2 and diastole. Both heart sound localization and segmentation can be divided into direct and indirect approaches. *Indirect methods* (section 4.2) exploit multimodal sensor information such as ECG and/or carotid pulse tracings [134], while *direct methods* (section 4.3) are operating solely on the PCG signal.

The most robust automatic segmentation methods are based on ECG-gating and are thus indirect. ECG-gating means that temporal information from the ECG is used to segment the PCG signal into heart cycles [134]. This is very convenient since the QRS complexes in the ECG are fairly easy to detect automatically. Since the heart sounds occur in certain time intervals after the QRS complex, the detection procedure is immensely facilitated. For example, finding S1 in a narrow search window where we know that it exists (but we do not know its exact location) is much easier than finding S1 in a larger search window where there might be multiple occurrences of S1 as well as S2 or other signal components. ECG based heart sound segmentation is addressed in section 4.2. In some cases, when it is important to find the boundaries of a heart sound accurately, manual segmentation by a phonocardiography expert is a viable alternative. Both multisensor data and denoising techniques may then be used to facilitate the manual segmentation process.

A related topic to ECG-gated heart sound segmentation is accurate localization of S1. The QRS complex is here regarded as a trigger for S1, making it possible to use event related ensemble averaging for noise reduction [15]. Very accurate localization of S1 is necessary in certain clinical situations where the timing of events is important. Measuring the fluctuations in cardiac time intervals is one such application which will be discussed in chapter 7. The ensemble averaging method for accurate S1 localization will be addressed in section 4.2.1.

Table 4.1: Time and frequency properties for the heart sounds.

Sound	Location (ms)	Duration (ms)	Freq. range (Hz)
S1	10–50 after R-peak in ECG	100–160	10–140
S2	280–360 after R-peak in ECG	80–140	10–400
S3	440–460 after R-peak in ECG or 120-180 after closure of semilunar valves	40–80	15-60
S4	40–120 after beginning of P-wave in ECG	30–60	15–45

Direct heart sound segmentation without the aid of an ECG is more complicated. The most important step in direct heart sound localization is to find a transform that takes the signal into a domain where S1 and S2 are emphasized. Several choices of this transformation have been presented over the years. Shannon energy [138], homomorphic filtering [86], frequency analysis [112], entropy analysis [247] and recurrence time statistics [14] are a few examples. After the transformation, a threshold is applied to locate the heart sounds. In section 4.3, several of these transforms will be presented and compared, using simulated data as well as experimental recordings. The basic concepts of direct heart sound segmentation are introduced in section 4.4.

The focus of this chapter is on finding either S1 or S2. However, detection of S3 is briefly discussed in section 4.5.

4.1 Properties of heart sounds

In healthy subjects, the frequency spectrum of S1 contains a peak in the low frequency range ($10 - 50$ Hz) and in the medium frequency range ($50 - 140$ Hz) [250]. S2 contains peaks in low- ($10 - 80$ Hz), medium- ($80 - 220$ Hz) and high-frequency ranges ($220 - 400$ Hz) [249]. S2 is composed of two components, one originating from aortic valve closure and one originating from pulmonary valve closure. Normally, the aortic component (A2) is of higher frequency than the pulmonary component (P2) [171]. The peaks probably arise as a result of the elastic properties of the heart muscle and the dynamic events that cause the various components of S1 and S2 [249,250]. S3 and S4 are believed to originate from vibrations in the left ventricle and surrounding structures powered by the acceleration and deceleration of blood flow. 75% of the total energy in S3 is contained below 60 Hz [144] while S4 mainly contain frequencies below 45 Hz [21]. The time and frequency properties of heart sounds are summarized in table 4.1 and examples of two phonocardiographic (PCG) signals and their frequency spectra are illustrated in figure 4.1.

There is a small delay between the aortic component and the pulmonary component causing a splitting of S2 (since right ventricular ejection terminates after left ventricular ejection). Normally, the splitting increases with inspiration due to increased blood return to the right heart, increased vascular capacitance of the pulmonary bed and decreased blood return to the left heart [226]. In certain heart diseases, this splitting can become wide, fixed or reversed (see further chapter 2). FFT analysis does

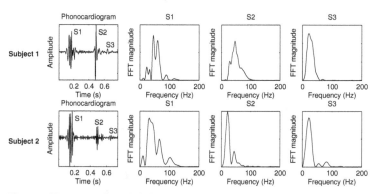

Fig. 4.1: **Heart sounds and their respective frequency spectra from a 13 year old girl (top row) and a 36 year old male (bottom row). Data obtained from data set VI.**

not take timing into consideration, so it cannot reveal which of the two valves closes first. Meanwhile, it is hard to notice any difference between the two components in the time domain. A tool able to investigate how the signal's frequency content varies over time is thus called for. An example showing the four heart sounds is presented in figure 4.2. Note that the two components of S2 are merged, but that the higher frequency aortic component precedes the lower frequency pulmonary component.

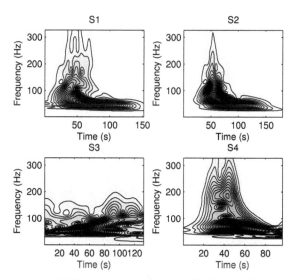

Fig. 4.2: **Example of TFR contour plots of S1, S2, S3 and S4 (note the different scaling of the x-axis). The S-transform was used to calculate the joint time-frequency distributions. Data obtained from data set VI.**

97

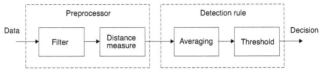

Fig. 4.3: Block diagram of a typical change detection setup. Figure adopted from Gustafsson [87].

4.2 Indirect heart sound localization and segmentation

S1 marks the onset of systole while S2 occurs at the start of diastole. The timing of the sounds is thus related to ventricular depolarization and repolarization (section 2.1.3). Hence, the ECG provides information about where to search for heart sounds (S1 occurs subsequent to the QRS complex and S2 occurs after the T-wave). This procedure is often referred to as *ECG-gating*. QRS detection algorithms basically follow a detector structure as outlined in figure 4.3. The purpose of each processing block (within the ECG setting) is summarized below:

- The *filter* suppresses noise and unwanted ECG components such as the P-wave and the T-wave. This is typically implemented with a bandpass filter (center frequency $10 - 24$ Hz, bandwidth $5 - 10$ Hz).

- Transformation of the signal into a domain where QRS complexes are emphasized provides a *distance measure* which maximizes the distance between the QRS complex and other signal components. The transformation is typically rectification, squaring or differentiation.

- The *detection rule* might be broken down into averaging and thresholding. Averaging is performed to ensure reasonable waveform duration and some robustness to noise. The threshold decides whether a new QRS complex has been found.

More information about ECG signal processing and robust QRS detection algorithms can be found in Sörnmo et al. [217] or Köhler et al. [125]. Based on the ECG signal, predefined search windows are used to locate the heart sounds, see figure 4.4. A typical window choice for S1 detection is $0.05RR - 0.2RR$, and for S2 detection, $1.2RT - 0.6RR$, where RR is the interval between two R-peaks and RT is the time interval from the R-peak to the T-wave [62]. How to actually find the heart sounds within these windows can be accomplished in several ways. Looking for the maximum value in the selected window is one (rather naive) approach, and looking at the time varying spectral content is another. ECG-gating in combination with Shannon energy will be used as a preprocessing step in sections 5.1 and 5.3. A thorough survey of different techniques able to emphasize heart sound occurrences in the PCG signal will be presented in section 4.3.

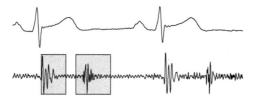

Fig. 4.4: **Example of ECG-gating with defined search windows for S1 and S2, respectively.**

4.2.1 Accurate localization of S1

In some applications, such as when deriving cardiac time intervals (chapter 7), very accurate temporal localization of the heart sounds is necessary [15]. The morphology of S2 varies a lot with respiration, so averaging over many heart cycles is inappropriate for noise reduction. In contrast to S2, the appearance of S1 changes little over time. Furthermore, S1 is event-related and occurs within a fairly constant time interval after the QRS complex in the ECG. These properties make S1 a perfect candidate for ensemble averaging (see section 3.7.1). An example showing S1 before and after denoising by ensemble averaging can be seen in figure 4.5. The noise reduction abilities of ensemble averaging rest upon a number of assumptions [217], whose validity in the PCG setting should be commented.

1. *The noise should be zero mean.* Since the PCG signal is a time series measuring vibrations on the body surface, the DC level is irrelevant. High pass filtering the signal or subtracting its mean is thus a safe operation which does not influence the frequency content of the heart sounds.

2. *The noise should be uncorrelated* from heart cycle to heart cycle. This is usually the case, but power line interference could present a problem. This interference has a frequency content of 50 or 60 Hz which overlaps the frequency content of the heart sounds. Possible solutions include notch-filters or estimation-subtraction methods [217].

3. *The morphology of S1 should be fixed* from heart cycle to heart cycle. This means that the alignment should be perfect and that the shape and width of S1 should be constant. It has been argued that ensemble averaging is inappropriate for noise reduction of PCG signals since the morphology of heart sounds varies with physiological processes such as respiration [93]. However, these variations in morphology mostly affect S2 while the appearance of S1 is quite robust. Averaging techniques such as dynamic time warping or integral shape averaging [34], which are able to compensate for time shifts and time scale fluctuations, might however improve the S1 template.

4. *There should be no correlation between signal and noise.* Most noise sources are additive and in these cases there are no correlations between the PCG signal

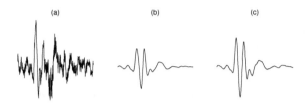

Fig. 4.5: Example of one realization of S1 (a) and the effect of denoising by ensemble averaging (b). The same example but derived with latency-corrected ensemble averaging is also illustrated (c). The lower amplitude in (b) is due to smearing since the time interval between the R-peak and S1 is not entirely constant. Figure adapted from Ahlstrom et al. [15].

and the noise. However, cardiac vibrations as well as other sound sources such as respiratory, muscle and abdominal noise are mixed in the thorax on their way to the body surface. This interaction probably causes correlations between the signal and some of the noise sources.

5. *The statistical distribution of the noise should be Gaussian.* Ensemble averaging is an optimal estimator if the noise is Gaussian, however, some results indicate that the noise distribution is slightly subgaussian in PCG signals [247]. This implies that a more robust averaging technique such as using the median instead of the mean might be beneficial.

Due to these issues, denoising by ensemble averaging might not be optimal. Nonetheless, ensemble averaging provides very good results when used for accurate S1 localization [15]. Following the approach outlined in Ahlstrom et al [15], we assume that each realization of S1, $x_i(t)$, is additively composed of random noise, $v_i(t)$, and a deterministic signal component, $S_1(t)$, see equation 4.1. The signal component is allowed to be shifted in time, and this latency shift is accounted for by the random variable θ_i.

$$x_i(t) = S_1(t - \theta_i) + v_i(t) \qquad (4.1)$$

The ensemble is constructed by cutting out the different realizations $x_i(t)$ from the PCG signal, using a 250 ms window starting with the R-peak in the ECG, see figure 4.6. To get an initial estimate of $S_1(t)$, a constant time delay between the R-peak and S1 is assumed. The maximum likelihood estimator of $S_1(t)$, assuming fixed white Gaussian noise, will then result in the estimated $\hat{S}_1(t)$, see equation 4.2, or its recursive counterpart, see equation 4.3. Note that $1/M$ in equation 4.3 can be replaced by a forgetting factor to only incorporate the latest realizations in the estimate. Since the time delay between the R-peak and S1 is not entirely constant, the variable latency shifts have to be adjusted for. This can be done by Woody's algorithm [243]. After the estimate $\hat{S}_1(t)$ has been obtained, it can be used as a patient specific template. By cross-correlating the template with the PCG signal, an output with strongly pronounced peaks at each S1 occurrence is obtained, see figure 4.6.

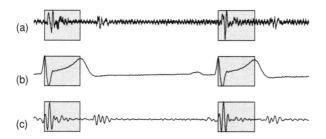

Fig. 4.6: Example of the original PCG signal (a), the ECG (b) and the output from cross-correlating the PCG signal with the template of S1 (c). The grey boxes indicate the time windows where S1 is sought for. Figure from Ahlstrom et al. [15].

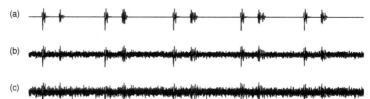

Fig. 4.7: Example showing a simulated PCG signal (a) and the same signal with an SNR of 0 dB and −5 dB, (b) and (c), respectively.

$$\hat{S}_1(t) = \frac{1}{M}\sum_{i=1}^{M} x_i(t) \tag{4.2}$$

$$\hat{S}_{1,M}(t) = \hat{S}_{1,M-1}(t)\frac{1}{M}\left(x_i(t) - \hat{S}_{1,M-1}(t)\right) \tag{4.3}$$

To evaluate an algorithm whose main purpose is to locate S1 accurately, it is necessary to test it on a signal where the true occurrences are known. Aiming at localization errors of just a few milliseconds, it is not feasible to use experimental data, even with an expert marking the heart sound occurrences. Instead, a simulated PCG signal (section 2.6) with known S1 occurrences can be created. Here we simulated a PCG signal with 500 heart cycles, drenched in white Gaussian noise corresponding to an SNR of −20, −15, −10 and −5 dB. An example of a simulated signal with additive noise is given in figure 4.7.

The denoising abilities of ensemble averaging can analyzed in a mean square error sense and as the percentage of correct detections. After only a few heart cycles, the localization algorithm provides excellent results at an SNR of −10 dB, see figure 4.8. At −15 dB, the algorithm stabilizes at a detection ratio of about 96% after 40 heart cycles. Corresponding values for −20 dB are 100 heart cycles and a detection rate of 45%. Similar convergence rates are also seen in the mean square error plot (figure 4.8).

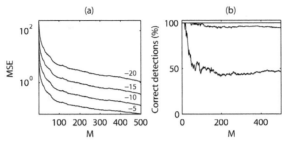

Fig. 4.8: Mean square error (MSE) as a function of the number of heart cycles (M) used in the calculation of $\hat{S}_1(t)$ (a). The different lines correspond to an SNR of -20, -15, -10 and -5 dB (top to bottom). Also shown is the percentage of correct detections as a function of the number of heart cycles used for noise reduction (b). The different lines correspond to an SNR of -20, -15, -10 and -5 dB (bottom to top, -10 and -5 dB are on top of each other). Figure from Ahlstrom et al. [15].

For comparison, the ensemble averaging algorithm can be compared with a multi-resolution approach [13]. This other algorithm operates according to the following steps:

1. Emphasize S1 occurrences by wavelet denoising (4th level Daubechies 6th wavelet using Stein's unbiased estimate of risk threshold, $f_s = 2$ kHz). Wavelet denoising is explained in section 3.7.2.

2. Segment the denoised PCG signal into cardiac cycles using the QRS complexes in the ECG signal.

3. Extract the envelope of the denoised PCG signal via the analytic signal. The analytic signal was explained in section 3.6.1.

4. Roughly locate S1 in each heart cycle as the maximum value in the envelope signal. This provides a coarse scale solution to the localization problem.

5. Derive a low-resolution (200 Hz low-pass filtered) and a high-resolution (400 Hz low-pass filtered) version of the denoised PCG.

6. Find the three largest peaks in the low-resolution signal in the vicinity of the coarse scale solutions. Select the first peak as the occurrence of S1. The reason for selecting several peaks is to increase robustness of the algorithm (due to noise, it is not obvious that the largest peak is the true peak).

7. Find the final localization solution by searching for a maximum in the high-resolution signal in the vicinity of the low-resolution solution.

The first step of this algorithm, wavelet denoising, may well be used in combination with ensemble averaging. In the following test, the above mentioned wavelet denoising scheme will be used as a preprocessing step before applying ensemble averaging. An example of the output from wavelet denoising and the consequent output after correlation with the ensemble averaged S1 template, applied to very noisy PCG data from one test subject in data set I, can be seen in figure 4.9.

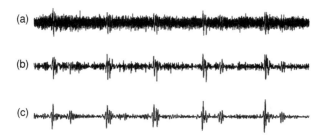

Fig. 4.9: Example of wavelet denoising (b) applied to a noisy PCG signal (a). After correlation with a template for S1, obtained with ensemble averaging, S1 is even further emphasized.

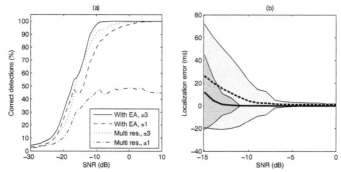

Fig. 4.10: The percentage of correct detections (a) and the localization error (b) as a function of signal to noise ratio. The different lines in (a) correspond to two error tolerances (±1 ms and ±3 ms, respectively) for the ensemble averaging (EA) approach and the multi resolution approach, respectively. In (b), the bold solid line and the dark grey area represent the $mean \pm std$ localization error for the ensemble averaging approach, while the bold dashed line and the light grey area show corresponding values for the multi resolution approach. Figure from Ahlstrom et al. [15].

The two S1 localization approaches were compared by Ahlstrom et al. [15]. A simulated signal with 1000 heart cycles was used, showing that very accurate results (95% correct detections with localization errors of less than ±1 ms) were obtainable for the ensemble averaging approach at an SNR of at least −3 dB, see figure 4.10. A corresponding value for an accuracy of ±3 ms was −10 dB. $\hat{S}_1(t)$ was then estimated recursively with $M = 20$. For the multi resolution approach, accurate results were obtainable at an SNR of -7 dB (±3 ms), while the best achievable detection rate was about 45% using an error tolerance of ±1 ms.

The two methods were also tested on experimental data containing a total amount of 11398 heart cycles (data set I). The number of correct S1 localizations was calculated via a trace of RS1-intervals. The RS1-interval was defined as the time duration between the R-peak in the ECG and S1, an interval with is is fairly constant between

Table 4.2: Correct S1 detections (%).

Subject	Multi resolution	Ensemble averaging
1	96.5	98.5
2	86.7	87.9
3	89.2	96.0
4	98.6	99.6
5	94.5	99.5
6	95.5	100
7	86.4	99.0
8	77.7	100
Mean±std	90.6 ± 7.1	97.6 ± 4.1

heart cycles. To get a quantitative measure of a correct S1 localization, detections that gave rise to RS1-intervals locally deviating more than three standard deviations from its neighboring RS1-intervals were considered erroneous. The running standard deviation was calculated in 5-second sliding windows. The RS1-traces were determined with the two S1 localization methods, and the averages used $M = 50$ heart cycles. To avoid unnecessary false detections close to the border of the signals, $\hat{S}_1(t)$ was estimated in a noncausal manner so that 50 heart cycles was always used in the estimation. The amounts of correct heart sound detections are presented in table 4.2.

The S1 template obtained by ensemble averaging can be used as a mother wavelet. Multiplying the template with a window function so that the endpoints are smoothly set to zero, both compact time support and differentiability are ensured. The template is also absolute and square integrable, thus fulfilling the basic conditions of a wavelet function. In Ahlstrom et al. [15], the template is only used as a matched filter. However, the next step would be to implement it as a patient-specific wavelet which is automatically adjusted to fit the signal at hand. Performing wavelet denoising with a customized mother wavelet would presumably increase the results further. A motivation for patient-specific studies is that the morphology of S1 differs a lot between patients. Based on the data in data set I, the cross-correlation coefficient between templates from different patients was found to vary from $0.26 - 0.81$. If the cross-correlation is as low as 0.26, it is not a very good idea to use the same analyzing function for all patients.

4.3 Direct heart sound localization

Heart sound localization algorithms operating solely on PCG data try to emphasize heart sound occurrences with an initial transformation. These transformations can roughly be classified into three main categories; frequency based transformations, morphological transformations and complexity based transformations. Most algorithms can be fitted into the detection scheme illustrated in figure 4.11, that is, filtering, applying a distance measure able to distinguish signal from noise, and smoothing and thresholding to separate signal from noise.

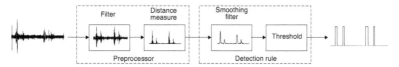

Fig. 4.11: Schematic description of heart sound localization. Noisy PCG data enters the filter where excessive noise is removed. The distance measure tries to maximize the distance between the heart sounds and the background noise, and the result is smoothed and thresholded.

4.3.1 Algorithm components

The frequency range of heart sounds is about $10 - 400$ Hz [249, 250]. Initial *filtering* can thus be used to remove excessive noise. A zero-phase low-pass filter with a cutoff frequency of 400 Hz will be used throughout this section. Some distance measures, particularly complexity based measures, make use of the less regular patterns in the noise to separate them from the signal. It could thus be advantageous to add a small amount of noise to the signal after filtering. An unfortunate trend in bioacoustic signal analysis suggests that the signals should be acquired at a very high sampling rate. The motivation is simply that nonlinear dynamic analysis tools show improved results when applied to densely sampled signals. This is, however, unnecessary. The damping of the signals as they pass through the thorax efficiently removes high frequency components why the higher sampling rate merely samples the noise more accurately. If high frequency noise is an inherent part of the analysis scheme, it is preferable to add it later in a more controlled manner. Throughout this section, a small amount of additive white Gaussian noise corresponding to an SNR of 30 dB will be added after the above mentioned filtering.

The *distance measure* is provided by the transformations mentioned in the beginning of this chapter. The main objective is to make the distance between signal and noise as large as possible. Many of the distance measures are operating on a batch of data. This processing is performed within a sliding window, resulting in a trace of calculated values over time. All traces will be normalized against the 99th percentile of their histograms. This approach is less sensitive to extreme values and outliers compared to normalizing against the maximum value of the feature trace. The traces are often somewhat jagged, why a *smoothing filter* may be applied. The smoothing filter is however method dependent and will be described in corresponding sections (4.3.4–4.3.6).

Another important design parameter is the *threshold*. A common threshold when looking for transient changes is the mean of the calculated trace plus its standard deviation according to equation 4.4. This approach will be used throughout this section, however, the mean value will be subtracted from the trace thus reducing the threshold to $\alpha \cdot \sigma_{trace}$.

$$\text{Threshold} = \mu_{trace} + \alpha \cdot \sigma_{trace} \tag{4.4}$$

4.3.2   Evaluation data

Both simulated and experimental data will be used to evaluate the algorithms. Design parameters and noise robustness will be evaluated on simulated data, while the methods' suitability for clinical use will be evaluated on experimental data. A simulated PCG signal (section 2.6) consisting of 100 heart cycles and white Gaussian noise, sampled at 2 kHz, will be used in the simulations. Some of the results from the simulation study will be presented along with the method descriptions in sections 4.3.4–4.3.6. This includes the determination of window size, threshold, positive and negative predictive values as a function of SNR and receiver operating characteristic curves. All signal examples in figures 4.13–4.26 are based on the simulated sound signal. Remaining simulation results will be presented in section 4.3.8.

The experimental data was chosen from 25 test subjects or patients with five different sources of noise in data sets IV and V on page 6. The chosen data set consists of 68 heart sounds from five test subjects during breath hold (from data set V), 90 heart sounds recorded from five test subjects during tidal breathing (from data set V), 115 heart sounds recorded from five test subjects during forced respiration (from data set V), 75 heart sounds recorded from five patients with severe aortic stenosis (from data set IV) and 75 heart sounds recorded from five patients with severe mitral insufficiency (MI, from data set IV). An example of the simulated PCG signal at different noise levels was shown in figure 4.7, while examples of real data from the five different groups are shown in figure 4.12. Manual segmentation aided by ECG data is used to find the true boundaries of the heart sounds in the experimental data set. Results from the experimental data set are presented in section 4.3.8.

4.3.3   Determination of design parameters

The two design parameters *threshold* and *window length* are very important for the results. In this section, the sliding window will be shifted by 5 ms, and each calculated value will be assigned to the midpoint of the window. The length of the window is a compromise where short windows give many false positives while long windows give smooth traces with many false negatives. Similarly, a low threshold provides many correct detections but also a lot of false detections, while higher thresholds might miss many heart sound occurrences. To find optimal values of the threshold and the window size, a global search was conducted. The optimum was determined via the product of negative predictive values and positive predictive values by maximizing the surface spanned by different window sizes and thresholds. The product between positive and negative predictive values gives high output when the two error measures are high and a low output if either or both of the measures are low.

Some methods operate on a sample-per-sample basis, rendering the window size inapplicable in the optimization procedure. In these cases, α was determined as the crossing between the positive and negative predictive value curves as they were plotted as a function of α. The smoothing filter and other method specific design parameters will be described in their corresponding sections (4.3.4–4.3.6).

106

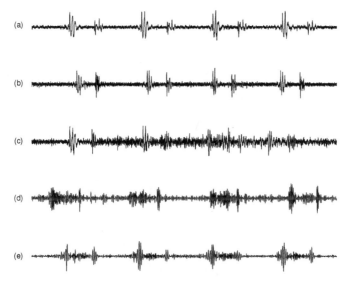

Fig. 4.12: **Examples of typical PCG signals from the data set used in the evaluation of heart sound localization algorithms. Signals acquired from test subjects during breath hold (a), tidal breathing (b) and forced respiration (c) as well as from patients with aortic stenosis (d) and mitral insufficiency (e).**

4.3.4 Frequencies and wavelets

The acoustic energy of S1 and S2 is mainly located in the frequency ranges $10 - 140$ Hz [250] and $10 - 400$ Hz [249], respectively. It is thus expected that the spectral content in the PCG signal, measured over time in the range $20 - 300$ Hz, will contain more energy at time instants where heart sounds are present [189]. Measuring the energy intensity in this range with the spectrogram is called the *average power method* for heart sound localization [189]. An intricate adaptive threshold based on the power of inspiratory and expiratory lung sounds and a patient specific adjustment parameter has been suggested for this method [189]. Here, the threshold was simply set according to equation 4.4. An example from the simulation study along with results from the simulation study are shown in figure 4.13. The design parameters of the algorithm were determined using figure 4.13b and set according to table 4.3 on page 118. From the figure, based on the positive and negative predictive values, it can be seen that the method stabilized at an SNR of -7 dB. The area under the ROC curve (at $SNR = 0$ dB) was found to be 0.90.

The *average power wavelet coefficient method* is an extension to the average power method. The main differences are that the spectrogram is calculated on the fifth approximation level of a Daubechies 4th wavelet ($f_s = 10$ kHz), that the intensity is calculated in the range $20-40$ Hz and that the threshold is calculated automatically

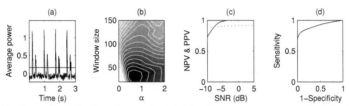

Fig. 4.13: Example of the time trace calculated by the average power method for four heart cycles (a). Results from a simulated signal ($SNR = -3$ dB) showing negative predictive value (NPV) multiplied with positive predictive value (PPV) for different window sizes and thresholds (α) are shown in (b), where dark colors indicate high performance values. Results showing PPV (solid line) and NPV (dotted line) as a function of SNR are shown in (c). A ROC curve ($SNR = 0$ dB) is shown in (d).

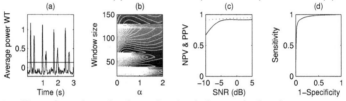

Fig. 4.14: Example and results from the simulation study for the average power wavelet coefficient method. See figure 4.13 for details regarding the subplots.

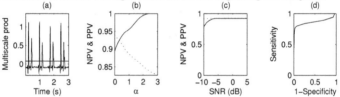

Fig. 4.15: Example of the time trace calculated by the multiscale product method for four heart cycles (a). Results from a simulated signal ($SNR = -3$ dB) showing negative predictive value (NPV, dotted line) and positive predictive value (PPV, solid line) for different thresholds are shown in (b) while results showing PPV and NPV as a function of SNR are shown in (c). A ROC curve ($SNR = 0$ dB) is shown in (d).

as the mean value of the energy of the noise [189]. Results from the simulation study are shown in figure 4.14. The method stabilized at an SNR of -5 dB and the area under the ROC curve (at $SNR = 0$ dB) was found to be 0.96. Using a low-frequency band for segmentation purposes has also been described by Haghighi-Mood et al. [92]. However, their work is based on ECG-gating as well as multiple acoustical sensors.

In the wavelet approaches, methods suggested throughout the literature specify a particular mother wavelet which should be used at a particular approximation or detail. These specifications are, however, dependent on the sampling frequency. Conversion to a more appropriate scale was done according to equation 4.5, where F_a is the pseudo frequency at scale a that we want to preserve, F_c is the center frequency of the wavelet and f_s is the sample frequency. The most suitable approximation or detail was then chosen based on the extracted center frequency.

$$F_a = \frac{F_c \cdot f_s}{a} \tag{4.5}$$

The product of adjacent wavelet decompositions can be used for noise reduction as well as for emphasizing singular signal components. The underlying principle is that Gaussian noise decreases while singular components increases when different scales are multiplied [20]. In the setting of heart sound localization, this property of multiscale products is very interesting since the "singular" heart sound will be emphasized while the noise level is reduced. This understanding is the reasoning behind the *multiscale product method* [68], where the product of the first three approximation levels of the Symlet wavelet (order 5) is calculated. An appropriate threshold can be set at the mean value plus five times the standard deviation of the PCG signal where heart sound segments have been removed [68]. The multiscale product often resulted in a jagged trace, why a smoothing filter (5th order zero phase Butterworth low-pass filter with a cut-off frequency of 20 Hz) was applied. An example of the multiscale product method is shown in figure 4.15. The method stabilized at an SNR of -7 dB and the area under the ROC curve (at $SNR = 0$ dB) was found to be 0.84.

A somewhat different approach towards extracting interesting signal components based on frequency behavior is *homomorphic filtering*. Assuming that the heart sounds are approximately amplitude modulated while murmurs and other sounds are either frequency modulated or both amplitude and frequency modulated, the two modulations can be separated by mapping the (multiplicative) signal into an additive domain. Hence, assume that the slowly varying heart sound envelope $l(t)$ is multiplied with a higher frequency signal $h(t)$. By taking the logarithm of the signal, equation 4.6, the non-linear multiplication changes into a linear addition, equation 4.7. The low frequency contribution $l(t)$ may then be extracted from the high frequency contribution $h(t)$ by a low-pass filter. Exponentiation takes the result back to the original signal domain, equation 4.8. If the low-pass filter is properly chosen, $l(t)$ will be a good estimate of the envelope.

$$
\begin{align}
s(t) &= l(t)h(t) \tag{4.6}\\
\ln s(t) &= \ln l(t) + \ln h(t) \tag{4.7}\\
e^{LP(\ln l(t) + \ln h(t))} &= e^{LP(\ln l(t)) + LP(\ln h(t))} \approx e^{LP(\ln l(t))} \approx l(t) \tag{4.8}
\end{align}
$$

An advantage with homomorphic filtering is its scalable smoothness, which handles the problem of S2 splits and serrated peaks by adjusting the low-pass filter [75]. The suggested threshold for the homomorphic filtering technique is to multiply the maximal value of the extracted envelope by a factor of 0.35 [86]. An example of the homomorphic filtering method applied to the simulated PCG signal is shown in figure 4.16. In this section, a 5th order Butterworth low-pass filter with a cut-off frequency of 20 Hz was used to extract the envelope. The method stabilized at an SNR of -4 dB and the area under the ROC curve (at $SNR = 0$ dB) was found to be 0.91.

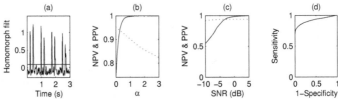

Fig. 4.16: Example and results from the simulation study for the homomorphic filtering method. See figure 4.15 for details regarding the subplots.

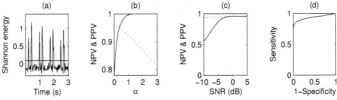

Fig. 4.17: Example and results from the simulation study for the Shannon energy method. See figure 4.15 for details regarding the subplots.

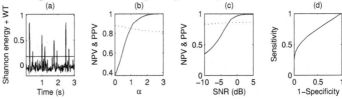

Fig. 4.18: Example and results from the simulation study for the Shannon entropy method applied to a wavelet detail. See figure 4.15 for details regarding the subplots.

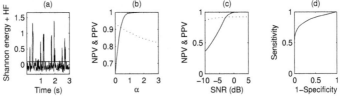

Fig. 4.19: Example and results from the simulation study for the homomorphic filtering method applied to the Shannon energy of a PCG signal. See figure 4.15 for details regarding the subplots.

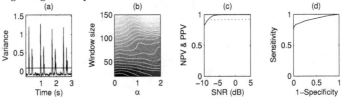

Fig. 4.20: Example and results from the simulation study for the variance method. See figure 4.13 for details regarding the subplots.

4.3.5 Quadratic measures

The quadratic measures operate on the signal's amplitude at a sample-per-sample basis. Since the amplitude enters the equations twice, these nonlinear techniques are related to the instantaneous energy of a signal. While the energy, equation 4.9, will bury low intensity sounds under high intensity ones, the *Shannon energy*, equation 4.10, will emphasize medium intensities and attenuate low intensities. This property is highly useful in emphasizing heart sounds, especially when murmurs are not present [138]. An example of Shannon energy applied to simulated PCG data is shown in figure 4.17. Shannon energy can be calculated in a sliding window, where each window is assigned an averaged measure [138]. However, when the overlap between consecutive windows is large, it is more efficient to calculate sample-per-sample values and smooth the results with a moving average filter. In this section, a 5th order zero phase Butterworth low-pass filter with a cut-off frequency of 30 Hz was used to extract the envelope. The method stabilized at an SNR of -4 dB and the area under the ROC curve (at $SNR = 0$ dB) was found to be 0.93.

$$\text{Energy } E(t) = s^2(t) \tag{4.9}$$

$$\text{Shannon energy } E(t) = -s^2(t) \cdot \log s^2(t) \tag{4.10}$$

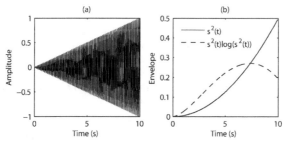

Fig. 4.21: Comparison of different envelope estimation methods. The test signal is presented in (a) and the smoothed results are shown in (b). The test signal was a 200 Hz sinusoid with amplitude ranging from 0 to 1 and sampled with 10 kHz. In this comparison, the output was low-pass filtered by a 5th order Butterworth filter with a cut off frequency of 150 Hz.

Two extensions have been suggested to the Shannon energy method. The first approach is to apply Shannon energy to the sixth detail of a Daubechies 6th wavelet ($f_s = 2$ kHz, [139]) and the second approach is to apply homomorphic filtering to the Shannon energy of the PCG signal [75]. Examples of these approaches are illustrated in figures 4.18 and 4.19. The same smoothing filter as in the original Shannon energy method was applied. The wavelet extension stabilized at an SNR of -2 dB and the area under the ROC curve (at $SNR = 0$ dB) was found to be 0.71. For the homomorphic extension, the corresponding results were -2 dB and 0.87, respectively.

4.3.6 Complexity based measures

Complexity is insensitive to absolute measures such as amplitude and frequency, and it has been claimed that this new family of features present a paradigm shift in biomedical signal analysis [197]. Complexity is an intuitive measure. When quantifying PCG signals, normal heart sounds have a certain structure whereas murmurs are more complex and background noise has no structure at all [95, 166]. Heart sound localization should hence be feasible by quantifying the amount of complexity in the PCG signal over time. Approaches for calculating complexity include descriptive statistics, entropy and fractal dimensions.

Running variance is a very simple test for tracking changes in system dynamics [87]. In the bioacoustic setting, the onset of a heart sound can be modeled as such a change in dynamics. However, since the DC level of a PCG signal is zero, the variance calculation collapses into a measure of average energy – a measure we opposed in the last paragraphs since it buries low intensity signal components under high intensity components. Nonetheless, a *variance based method* for emphasizing heart sounds has been suggested [163], and a signal example along with simulation results are shown in figure 4.20. The method stabilized at an SNR of -7 dB and the area under the ROC curve (at $SNR = 0$ dB) was found to be 0.90.

A Gaussian distribution can be fully described by its second order moments (mean, variance and autocorrelation), leaving the higher order moments equal to zero. This implies that, as long as the interesting signal components are not Gaussian, efficient change detection algorithms can be developed which are very robust to Gaussian noise. The third and fourth order correspondences to variance are skewness and kurtosis, respectively. An example of a *kurtosis based method* for heart sound localization is illustrated in figure 4.22. The kurtosis method stabilized at an SNR of -2 dB and the area under the ROC curve (at $SNR = 0$ dB) was found to be 0.84. In contrast to skewness, kurtosis allows asymmetric distributions, making it a better choice for heart sound localization.

Variance and kurtosis are two features that stem from the theory of stochastic processes. An alternative way to conceptualize complexity is to plunge into the theory of dynamical systems. Here the system can be characterized by invariant measures such as fractal dimensions or entropy. There are two main approaches to estimate these invariants; those that operate directly on the waveform[1] and those that operate in a reconstructed state space.

Entropy can be interpreted as the average rate at which predictability is lost, and is thus a measure of system regularity [198]. There are several methods available for entropy estimation, and a suitable choice for heart sound localization is the *Shannon entropy* [247], see equation 4.11. Note the difference between this definition of Shannon entropy (which is applied to the probability density function) and the Shannon energy which was used to estimate the envelogram on a sample-per-sample

---

[1]Many waveform approaches are, strictly speaking, also stochastic in their nature [197].

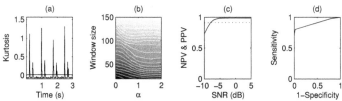

Fig. 4.22: Example and results from the simulation study for the kurtosis method. See figure 4.13 for details regarding the subplots.

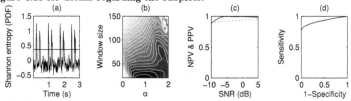

Fig. 4.23: Example and results from the simulation study for the Shannon entropy method, operating on the probability density function of the signal. See figure 4.13 for details regarding the subplots.

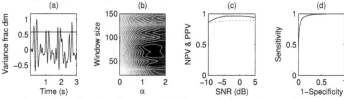

Fig. 4.24: Example and results from the simulation study for the variance fractal dimension method. Since the mean value of the fractal dimension trace was subtracted, the signal is not limited to $1 \geq dim \geq 2$. See figure 4.13 for details regarding the subplots.

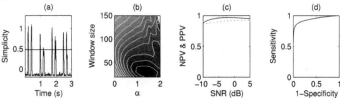

Fig. 4.25: Example and results from the simulation study for the simplicity method. See figure 4.13 for details regarding the subplots.

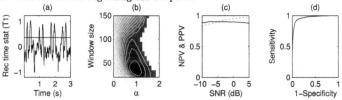

Fig. 4.26: Example and results from the simulation study for the recurrence time statistics method. See figure 4.13 for details regarding the subplots.

basis in section 4.3.5.

$$H(p) = -\sum_{i=1}^{N} p(i) \log p(i) \tag{4.11}$$

Entropy calculations can be done in both the reconstructed state space and on the waveform. In the reconstructed state space, the probability density function will be of the same dimensionality as the embedding space. A lot of data is thus required when estimating these high dimensional probability density functions. In the application of heart sound localization, the sliding window provides an upper limit to the amount of data that can be used. State space based entropy measures are thus out of the question. The probability density function may also be estimated directly from the PCG signal to obtain a waveform entropy estimate. An example of Shannon entropy from the simulation study is shown in figure 4.23. The waveform Shannon entropy stabilized at an SNR of -7 dB and the area under the ROC curve (at $SNR = 0$ dB) was found to be 0.92. Even when operating on the waveform, the amount of data in a short window, 20 ms in this section, might not be enough. To increase the accuracy of the probability density estimate, it is possible to replace the classic histogram with improved kernel based estimators, see equation 4.12, where K is the kernel, h is the kernel bandwidth, N is the number of observations $s(i)$ and $\hat{p}_i(S)$ is the estimated probability density function. In Yadollahi et al. [247], a normal kernel $K(S) = (1/2\pi)e^{-S^2/2}$ was used with the kernel bandwidth $h = 1.06\hat{\sigma}(S)N^{-0.2}$, where $\hat{\sigma}$ is the standard deviation of the input observations.

$$\hat{p}_i(S) = \frac{1}{N} \sum_{i=1}^{N} \frac{1}{h} K\left(\frac{S - s(i)}{h}\right) \tag{4.12}$$

Another complexity measure is the fractal dimension, a statistical quantity that conveys information on spatial extent (convolutedness or space filling properties), self similarity (the ability to remain unchanged when the scale of measurement is changed) and self-affinity (different scaling properties in different directions). Calculating the fractal dimension in a reconstructed state space requires a lot of data, why this approach was not applicable in the heart sound localization application (due to the sliding window approach). In waveform fractal dimension analysis, the signal is looked upon as a planar set in $\mathbb{R}^2$ where the dimension is a measure of the signal's spatial extent. Note that the waveform fractal dimension is measured in $\mathbb{R}^2$ and thus limited to the range $1 \leq dim \leq 2$, and that it normally differs from the dimension of the attractor (measured in the reconstructed state space). There are several methods available for waveform fractal dimension estimation; the *variance fractal dimension* [124] and *Katz waveform fractal dimension* [120] are two of them. The variance fractal dimension was used in this section, and a signal example along with simulation results are illustrated in figure 4.24. A dyadic time increment was used since it is preferable for separating signal components [124]. The variance fractal dimension stabilized at an SNR of -5 dB and the area under the ROC curve (at $SNR = 0$ dB) was found to be 0.97. Since heart sounds have a lower fractal dimension compared to background noise [95, 166], the fractal dimension trace was inverted to get peaks at each heart sound occurrence instead of valleys. No particular threshold has been reported for this technique [76].

114

So far, only waveform measures of complexity have been considered. We will now look at two methods operating in the reconstructed state space. Both of these methods have been developed to be applicable to short data sets, turning them into suitable candidates for heart sound localization algorithms. The first method is based on singular spectrum analysis [197] and the second method is based on recurrence time statistics [73]. Heart sounds have a characteristic appearance in state space, see figure 4.27, therefore it is not surprising that state space approaches are suitable for heart sound localization. Some additional design parameters are necessary in these two algorithms; the time delay τ and the embedding dimension d. How to choose these parameters properly was described in section 3.4.

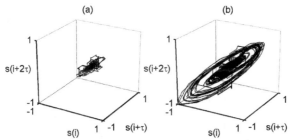

Fig. 4.27: State space trajectories ($d = 3$, $\tau = 12$) of a PCG signal with heart sounds present (b) and with heart sounds removed (a). The transition between the two attractors is reflected in both the singular spectrum and in the recurrence time statistic, hence indicating when a heart sound is present. Figure from Ahlstrom et al. [14].

The complexity of the embedding matrix can be quantified through the eigenvalues of the correlation matrix $C = X^T X$, where X is the embedding matrix. If the embedding dimension d is chosen large enough so that redundancy arises, the rank of the embedding matrix is an upper bound to the trajectory dimension [197], a finding that can be used for estimating system complexity. More precisely, the Shannon entropy of the normalized eigenvalues is calculated and the complexity value is determined as two to the power of the entropy. An embedding dimension of $d = 6$ and a time delay of $\tau = 1$ are suitable to create the embedding matrix [166], and a simulated signal example of the technique applied to heart sound localization can be seen in figure 4.25. This technique stabilized at an SNR of -5 dB and the area under the ROC curve (at $SNR = 0$ dB) was found to be 0.94.

Recurrence time statistics are sensitive to changes in system dynamics. There are two types of recurrence times, T1 and T2, where T1 is more robust to the noise level while T2 is preferable for detecting transitions with very low energy [73]. T1 is related to the information dimension via a power law, which motivates its ability to detect signal transitions based on signal amplitude, period, dimension and complexity [73]. In heart sound localization, the heart sounds represent a rather large transient change in the dynamics, why T1 was found to be the better choice in this application [14]. T1 basically measures the average amount of neighbors of an average state in state space. A parameter ε defines if two states are close enough to be neighbors, and can thus be seen as a filter. ε can be set adaptively using the running standard deviation of a high-pass filtered signal. A cut-off frequency of 300 Hz was used to filter out most of the heart sound energy, thus approximately setting ε to the variance of the noise. The embedding parameters were determined via auto mutual information and Cao's method, as outlined in section 3.4. Note that τ, d and ε were all set automatically. An example of T1 applied to the simulated heart sound signal is illustrated in figure 4.26. The T1 measure stabilized at an SNR of -1 dB and the area under the ROC curve (at $SNR = 0$ dB) was found to be 0.96.

4.3.7   Multi-feature heart sound localization

When comparing the simulation results from the last sections (summarized in table 4.4), it becomes clear that some methods are suitable for emphasizing heart sounds in certain situations while other methods are preferable in other situations. An obvious thought is then to combine the output from different methods to make use of their individual strengths. It would be possible to choose all the approaches in the previous section, however, due to the curse of dimensionality, a smaller subset of (preferably) independent features will be selected. Even though there are methods available to select the most efficient features (see section 3.10), a number of features will be picked more or less arbitrarily in this section. Based partly on intuition (trying to include features based on independent measures) and partly on results from the simulation study (excluding features with poor performance), the following feature set was investigated:

- Average power wavelet coefficient
- Shannon energy
- Variance
- Shannon entropy
- Variance fractal dimension
- Simplicity

The output from different methods and different patients have different amplitude ranges. Many classification techniques does however perform better when the features have similar dynamic range because of the way the thresholds are adapted in multiple dimensions. This can be achieved by normalizing the features. This is usually done by subtracting the mean and dividing by the standard deviation, but this approach is largely affected by the signal content. For instance, both the mean value and the standard deviation is larger in a feature trace where heavy respiration or murmurs are present. Instead, the feature traces can be normalized against the 99th percentile of their histograms. This approach is less sensitive to extreme values and outliers compared to normalizing against the maximum value of the feature trace.

A fully connected feed-forward neural network (sections 3.5 and 3.9), with logarithmic sigmoid transfer functions and biased values throughout was adopted to measure the performance of the combined feature set. Six input units were connected to two hidden layers, where the number of units in the first hidden layer was set to three.

The number of units in the second hidden layer was also set to three and the number of output units was set to one. The input to the network consisted of the traces from the six distance measures listed above. Each example presented to the network thus corresponded to the six trace values obtained at each time instant. An example showing the structure of the neural network is illustrated in figure 4.28. The target values were 0 (no heart sound) or 1 (heart sound). The network was thus set up for heart sound localization, where the aim is to find heart sounds, not to distinguish between the two. Since results from the simulation study was used for feature selection, only data from the experimental data set was used in the evaluation of the network.

The output from the network was thresholded at two times the standard deviation and compared to the manual segmentation results. A leave-one-out approach (section 3.11.1) was used for training and testing due to the limited amount of patients. Since data from all five groups of data were used in the training procedure, a general network was expected, able to handle signals recorded in many different situations (ranging from very noisy data covered in respiratory sounds to PCG signals recorded from patients with high intensity murmurs). If the minimum gradient was reached before the performance goal or the maximum number of epochs was reached, the training procedure was restarted with new initial conditions.

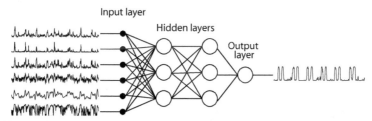

Fig. 4.28: Schematic description of the fully connected neural network with 6 inputs, 1 output and 3 + 3 neurons in the hidden layers. Transfer functions of logarithmic sigmoid type and biased values are used throughout.

4.3.8 Comparison between methods

Simulations

Thresholds and window sizes were determined using the simulated data, so it is not surprising that most methods performed well in the simulation study. In reality, the heart sounds do not behave as predictable as the simulated data indicates, and neither is the noise stationary nor entirely additive. The results from the simulation study should thus be interpreted with caution, and the simulations should mainly be seen as an approach to find proper values of the design parameters (table 4.3).

The global search for optimal parameter values, see figures 4.13–4.26, resulted in the parameters in table 4.3. The *average power wavelet coefficient* provided a very complicated parameter space, see figure 4.14, and it is likely that the chosen values are unstable. For *recurrence time statistics*, the maximum value indicated a window

Table 4.3: Design parameters for the different algorithms. The threshold is given as a multiple of the standard deviation ($\alpha \cdot \sigma$) of the PCG signal according to equation 4.4.

Method	Window length (ms)	Threshold
Average power	30	$0.8\,\sigma$
Average power WT	70	$0.5\,\sigma$
Multiscale products	—	$0.3\,\sigma$
Homomorphic filtering	—	$0.3\,\sigma$
Shannon energy (signal)	—	$0.3\,\sigma$
Shannon energy (signal) + WT	—	$0.9\,\sigma$
Shannon energy (signal) + HF	—	$0.35\,\sigma$
Variance	20	$0.4\,\sigma$
Kurtosis	20	$0.1\,\sigma$
Shannon entropy (PDF)	20	$1.0\,\sigma$
Variance fractal dimension	80	$1.5\,\sigma$
Simplicity	30	$1.5\,\sigma$
Recurrence time statistics (T1)	70	$0.8\,\sigma$

size of about 30 ms. However, this value was not chosen in favor of a larger window (70 ms) to provide more data for state space reconstruction. Some methods operate on a sample-per-sample basis, in these cases the window size was obviously left out of the optimization procedure.

Positive and negative predictive values were calculated as a function of SNR to investigate the robustness of the methods to noise (figures 4.13–4.26). It is evident that most methods do not perform well at an $SNR < -5$ dB.

The area under the ROC curve, at an $SNR = 0$ dB, for each method is shown in table 4.4. Three methods provided very good results, the *average power wavelet coefficient*, the *variance fractal dimension* and the *recurrence time statistic*. The two refinements of Shannon energy, see figures 4.19 and 4.18, provided the worst performance in the simulation study. It is interesting that these refinements performed worse than the original Shannon energy algorithm. A likely reason is that the wavelet detail of the PCG signal, even though it did emphasize the heart sounds, also reduced the medium amplitude components that are brought forward by Shannon energy, thus canceling out the expected performance gain. In the case of homomorphic filtering after applying the Shannon energy algorithm, difficulties arose when the signal was rectified by the quadratic transform, thus destroying the frequency modulated part of the signal which is one of the key components in homomorphic signal analysis.

Accurate localization of the heart sound boundaries is important in some applications such as heart sound cancellation (see chapter 6). Locating the onset of the sounds was easier compared to finding the slowly subduing endpoint of the sound waves, why the performance for endpoint detection was nearly one order of magnitude lower for most methods. Nonetheless, most methods provided very good boundary detection performance, finding both the onset and the endpoint of the

Table 4.4: Simulation results. Accuracy of onset and ending boundary detections, area under the ROC curve and processing time for a simulated signal with 100 heart cycles (74.1 s) at an $SNR = 0$ dB.

Method	Onset (ms)	Ending (ms)	AUC (%)	CPU time (ms)
Average power	6 ± 28	49 ± 37	90.1	2079
Average power WT	24 ± 50	34 ± 53	95.6	2371
Multiscale products	9 ± 5	45 ± 16	84.5	94
Homomorphic filtering	4 ± 3	42 ± 16	91.0	75
Shannon energy (signal)	6 ± 3	27 ± 15	92.6	340
Shannon energy (signal) + WT	144 ± 188	206 ± 212	71.3	340
Shannon energy (signal) + HF	14 ± 10	37 ± 15	86.8	342
Variance	3 ± 2	49 ± 37	89.6	861
Kurtosis	3 ± 2	49 ± 29	83.5	1216
Shannon entropy (PDF)	2 ± 2	36 ± 18	91.7	8740
Variance fractal dimension	160 ± 220	158 ± 228	96.8	7972
Simplicity	9 ± 28	46 ± 34	93.6	15791
Recurrence time statistics (T1)	24 ± 57	34 ± 60	95.6	46287

heart sounds with an error marginal of only a few hundreds of a second. In the simulation study, the *Shannon energy wavelet detail* and the *variance fractal dimension* performed considerably worse than the other methods.

The computational complexity of the methods is indicated in table 4.4. The absolute values of these measures are not very interesting, but it should be noted that some of the methods are really slow. Worst was the *recurrence time statistic* followed by other complexity based measures such as *simplicity, variance fractal dimension* and *Shannon entropy*. On the bright side, some of the top performers such as *average power wavelet coefficient* and the *Shannon energy* were really fast.

Experimental data

When so many contemporary approaches are available to solve the same task, it often implies that no good solution yet exists. Many methods in this section gave similar overall performance results, and all in all, the detection results were acceptable on low level noise data. However, results deteriorated in the presence of murmurs or forced respiration. To put it another way, no standard solution for direct heart sound localization is yet ready for clinical use.

The area under the ROC curves, see figure 4.29, indicated that the *variance fractal dimension* provided the best detection results closely followed by the *average power wavelet coefficient method* and *Shannon entropy*. The main performance difference became clear in the presence of MI where the *variance fractal dimension* was considerably better. Combining various methods in a *neural network* classifier did not improve the performance much. The distance between signal and noise was increased by the network, mostly by subduing the noise floor. However, this only applied to signals with low SNR. In presence of murmurs or heavy breathing, the output actually showed decreased performance compared to some of the features that were fed to the network.

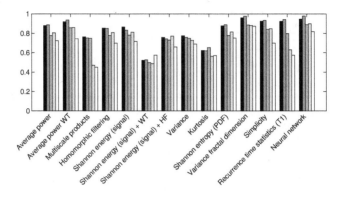

Fig. 4.29: Area under the ROC curve. The five bars in different shades of gray represents the five groups of experimental data; breath hold, tidal breathing, forced respiration, aortic valve stenosis and mitral insufficiency.

Both *Shannon energy* and *homomorphic filtering* showed a pretty good overall performance, however, the two refinements of these methods moved the ROC curves towards the diagonal. These results agreed with the simulation study. Again, the reason was that the wavelet detail used to bring out heart sounds and suppress noise, gave the heart sounds higher amplitudes which were dampened by the subsequent Shannon energy calculation. In the homomorphic filtering case, problems were introduced when the Shannon energy transform rectified the signal.

Interestingly, *variance* attained better test results as compared to *kurtosis*. The simulation study, where white Gaussian noise was added to a simulated PCG signal, was an ideal situation for the kurtosis method since kurtosis is zero for Gaussian data. Unfortunately, the heart sounds were nearly Gaussian themselves and therefore considerably dampened by the method. On the experimental data set, the rather noisy signal obstructed with forced respiration gave the best results when using the kurtosis method. Accurate results were expected since the respiratory signal is nearly Gaussian [247], but that the results should be worse on the other types of data came as a surprise. *Variance* on the other hand showed stable results across the different groups of experimental data.

The nonlinear complexity based measures *Shannon entropy, variance fractal dimension, simplicity* and *recurrence time statistics* all performed very well in the presence of respiratory noise. Indeed, all of these methods (except *simplicity*) were developed to operate on lung sound data where heart sounds are present, so the methods should be capable to handle this kind of data. The performance of the state space based approaches of *simplicity* and *recurrence time statistics* strongly deteriorated when applied to murmur data. In the MI group, the worst examples sometimes performed worse than chance (this was also the case for the *kurtosis, Shannon entropy, multiscale products* and the two refinements of Shannon energy). Possibly, the amount of data in the short sliding windows was enough to separate heart sounds from additive Gaussian noise as well as from respiratory noise, but not to distinguish different cardiac sounds from each other. Nevertheless, nonlinear analysis techniques still look promising for heart sound localization. For instance, the *variance fractal dimension* gave the best performance in the whole test.

4.4 Heart sound classification

So far, methods able to emphasize occurrences of heart sounds have been investigated. The final task would then be to label the detected peaks as S1, S2 or as a false detection. Lehner et al. proposed an indirect algorithm for PCG segmentation that estimates the onset of S1 with the QRS-complex in the ECG and the onset of S2 with the dicrotic notch in a carotid pulse tracing [134]. Other available approaches are based on segmenting the PCG signal into heart cycles using QRS-complexes followed by peak detection [92]. However, when an ECG (or other) recording is not available, other approaches are necessary. The most common direct technique is to use interval statistics [75, 138]:

1. Merge peaks that are very close (about $20ms$ apart).
2. If the peaks are too dispersed, lower the threshold and search for new local maxima.
3. Assign systole to short intervals which do not vary much over time.
4. Assign diastole to the remaining intervals.
5. Assign S1 or S2 labels to each peak so that S1 signals the start of systole and S2 the start of diastole.

The duration of systole and diastole is illustrated by the binominal distribution in figure 4.30. The duration of systole and diastole is also shown as a function of heart rate in figure 4.31. Clearly, classification algorithms associating the short time interval with systole runs into trouble with tachycardiac patients. Throughout this book, classification is dealt with using either ECG-gating or manual segmentation aided by an ECG. The main argument for using ECG-gating is the indisputable advantages when it comes to noise robustness and accuracy. For further details about direct heart sound classification, the reader is referred to the works by Liang et al. [138] and Gill et al. [75].

4.5 Finding the third heart sound

Heart sound localization usually deals with the task of finding S1 and S2. However, there might also be a third or a fourth heart sound (see chapter 2). Especially the third heart sound is clinically interesting due to its established connection with heart failure [158]. Compared to the task of locating S1 and S2, finding S3 is harder due to its low amplitude, short duration and low frequency [109]. The number of available methods for automatic S3 detection is very limited. One approach is to use a matched wavelet [108, 109] and another is based on the T2 statistic [10].

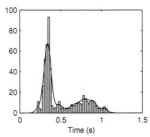

Fig. 4.30: Histogram of the density distribution of heart sound occurrences based on 273 heart cycles from the healthy subjects, i.e. the first three groups, in the experimental data set. It can be seen that systole (the first peak) is nearly constant and normally shorter than the duration of diastole (the second peak). The scaled kernel density estimate (equation 4.12) is also included in the figure.

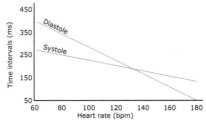

Fig. 4.31: Duration of systole and diastole as a function of heart rate. Note that the duration of diastole decreases heavily with increased heart rate while the duration for systole remains fairly constant. Redrawn from El-Segaier et al. [62].

The matched wavelet is defined as a band-pass Bessel filter, which is morphologically very similar to the third heart sound. The main idea is to decompose the PCG signal into four frequency bands corresponding to 17, 35, 60 and 160 Hz. The key observation behind the method is that S1 and S2 are present in all four frequency bands whereas S3 can only be found in the three lower bands. A detection algorithm is used to decide if a peak is present in a time window 130 ms after the heart sounds (no separate identification of S1 and S2 is made, so S3 has to be sought after both S1 and S2[2]). If a peak is detected in any of the 17, 35, 60 Hz bands and if the peak is large compared to the amplitudes found in the 160 Hz band, then an S3 occurrence is marked. The algorithm along with signal examples is shown in figure 4.32.

T1 was used in the previous section to locate S1 and S2. Here a related statistic, T2, is used for detection of S3. T1 is more robust to noise while T2 is more sensitive to changes in the signal. S3 is a very weak signal, so T2 statistics is the better choice here. T1 can thus be used to locate S1 and S2 whereas T2 can be used to detect S3. As in the matched wavelet approach, S3 is sought in a window after both S1 and S2. Selecting the proper neighborhood for determining if two neighbors

---

[2]This limitation can be avoided by inclusion of an ECG recording, making it easy to differentiate between S1 and S2.

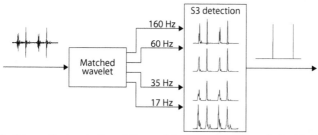

Fig. 4.32: Schematic description of the matched wavelet approach for S3 detection. The incoming PCG signal is decomposed into four frequency bands: 17, 35, 60 and 160 Hz, where peaks in the 60Hz band are assumed to be either S1 or S2. If a peak is present in a search window after S1 and S2 in either of the 17, 35, 60 bands, an S3 is assumed to be present. The output to the right in the figure indicates that two S3 occurrences were found in this example.

are close or not can be a problem. In figure 4.33, T1 and T2 are plotted for a range of ε-values to visualize their dependence on the neighborhood size. S1 and S2 are found using a simple threshold, but finding S3 (in T2) is somewhat harder. A whole range of ε-values can be calculated resulting in a T2-matrix, see figure 4.33. The resulting 2D-image can then be converted into 1D by an edge detection algorithm (implemented by low-pass filtering and detection of the maximum value in each column). In the 1D signal, an S3 occurrence is marked if a peak is present within the previously defined time window. The chosen detection rule compares the amplitude of the peak with the amplitude of the base line level [10].

In a comparison between the matched wavelet method and T2 method (on data set VI), the latter showed an improved detection rate, 98 % compared to 93 %. The increased detection rate came at the expense of more false detections, 7 % compared to 2 %. The lack of a proper analysis of the inherent thresholds, including receiver operating characteristics, is a major weakness in this comparison. However, combining the two methods, using T2 to locate S3 while the matched wavelet approach excludes false detections, could be a sound way to improve the results.

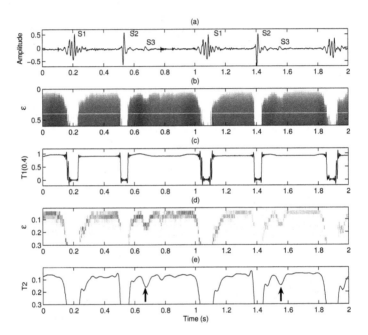

Fig. 4.33: Example of a PCG signal where S1, S2 and S3 are marked (a). T1, calculated for a range of ε-values, is shown in (b) while a single T1 is shown in (c) for $\varepsilon = 0.4$. $T1(0.4)$ is used to find S1 and S2. T2, calculated for a whole range of ε-values is shown in (d). An edge detection algorithm is used to convert T2 to the 1D signal in (e) which is used to detect S3 (marked as arrows by the detection algorithm).

5

Assessing and Classifying
Systolic Murmurs

"Take care of the sense, and the sounds will take care of themselves."
Lewis Caroll (1832–1898)

The main purpose of this chapter is to investigate whether information derived from a reconstructed state space can be used to assess and classify heart murmurs. Aortic stenosis (AS) will be investigated in section 5.1, mitral insufficiency (MI) will be investigated in section 5.2 and an attempt to classify innocent murmurs, murmurs caused by AS and murmurs caused by MI will be investigated in section 5.3.

Vibrations can be described by different time representations such as displacement (m), velocity (m/s) and acceleration (m/s^2). These classic PCG representations basically contain the same information, but for visual interpretation or time signal processing, they reveal different vibratory patterns [234]. Plotting these representations against each other, a reconstructed state space expressed in derivative coordinates is obtained, see figure 5.1. By observing the cardiohemic system via the PCG signal, the reconstructed state space is an attempt to recreate the dynamics of the flow (compare with figure 3.9). In this chapter, information extracted from the reconstructed state space will be investigated for murmur characterization.

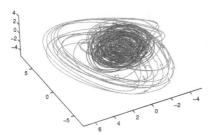

Fig. 5.1: Example of an embedded PCG signal. The heart sounds are encircling the more complex murmur.

125

5.1 Assessing and classifying systolic ejection murmurs

If the aortic or pulmonary valves become narrowed or constricted (stenotic), blood has to be forced through the valve opening. The arising turbulent blood flow causes vibrations in the cardiac structure which are perceived as murmurs. The murmur peaks in mid-systole at the time of maximal ejection and produces a crescendo-decrescendo shape in the PCG signal. As outlined in chapter 2, the severity of the stenosis influences the shape of the murmur, where the intensity will increase and the peak will occur later in systole as the stenosis becomes more severe. Since a boost from the atrium might be necessary to help build up the pressure in the ventricle, a fourth heart sound may be present. An ejection click may occur if the valves are brought to an abrupt halt instead of opening completely when moving from their closed position in diastole to their open position in systole. The appearances of murmurs caused by various degrees of AS are illustrated in figure 5.2.

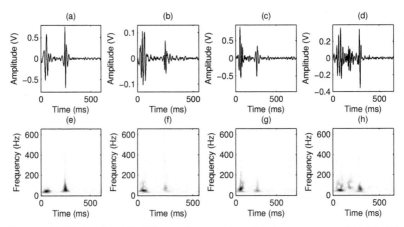

Fig. 5.2: **PCG signals with different degrees of aortic stenosis (group A1, A2, B1 and B2 in data set II with aortic flow velocities 1.55 m/s, 1.85 m/s, 3.2 m/s and 4.4 m/s in (a)–(d), respectively). Corresponding joint time-frequency representations are illustrated in (e)–(h). The grouping of data set II was defined on page 8. Note how difficult it is to distinguish murmurs in group A2 from murmurs in group B1.**

In pulmonic stenosis, a splitting in S2 is caused by increased capacitance in the dilated pulmonary trunk. In severe stenosis, S2 is widely split but difficult to hear since the pulmonary component is faint and the aortic component is obscured by the murmur. The degree of stenosis correlates well with the width of S2 [71]. The degree of pulmonic stenosis also correlates significantly with both the time interval from the cardiac electrical polarization to the ejection click and the location of peak amplitude of the systolic murmur [71].

In AS, there will be a paradoxical splitting of S2 that increases with expiration. If the stenosis is severe the aortic component is attenuated or even missing. Unfortunately, the width of the split is not significantly correlated with AS severity, and neither are variations in the peak amplitude of the murmur nor the timing of the ejection click [71].

The remainder of this section will deal with alternative methods to assess AS severity based on the PCG. Valvular disease is common in elderly humans. Mild sclerotic thickening of the aortic valves affect 25% of adults above 65 years, and the condition causes AS in 2% [219]. The clinical standard for diagnosing and quantifying AS severity is echocardiography, but it is often during auscultation that the disease is initially detected. Distinguishing heart murmurs caused by mild AS from innocent murmurs is a diagnostic challenge, and current murmur assessments as well as echocardiographic evaluations are sometimes inconclusive in these patients. Finding a simple and cost effective tool to find these patients during auscultation would thus be very valuable.

PCG based assessment of AS severity has previously been based on timing and frequency properties of the heart sounds and of the murmur. Classic time domain signatures include duration of the murmur, the timing of peak intensity of the systolic murmur and splitting of the second heart sound. However, according to Gamboa et al. [71], these are not convincing parameters. Spectral properties seem more reliable, and there is an established relationship between the murmur's frequency content and the severity of the stenosis [203]. For instance, the dominant frequency of the murmur has been related to the jet velocity distal to the stenosis [49], the percentage of higher frequencies has been related to transvalvular pressure differences [170] and a recent method, exploiting properties from joint time-frequency analysis, have found good correlations between the duration of higher frequency components and the peak pressure gradient [123]. In this section, properties going beyond linear approaches will be investigated. The 27 boxer dogs from data set II will be used for evaluation, and reported results are compiled from references [7], [101] and [8]. The statistical tests have been slightly changed compared to the original articles.

The features to be investigated are listed below. The cited references indicate where the feature was originally introduced for AS assessment.

1. Dominant frequency [49].
2. Duration of the murmur with frequency components above 200 Hz [123].
3. Murmur energy ratio [170].
4. Correlation dimension [101].
5. Sample entropy [8].
6. RQA – Recurrence rate [7].
7. RQA – Determinism [7].
8. RQA – Mean diagonal line length [7].
9. RQA – Max diagonal line length [7].
10. RQA – Entropy [7].
11. RQA – Laminarity [7].

12. RQA – Trapping time [7].

13. RQA – Max vertical line length [7].

5.1.1 Pre-processing

The PCG signals in data set II were segmented into S1, systole and S2 using ECG-gated Shannon energy. The local maxima of the PCG signal's envelope within pre-defined time windows were determined as S1 and S2, and the first local minima before and after S1 and S2 were used to determine the boundaries of the heart sounds. The region of interest in this study, focusing on the systolic period, was defined as the start of S1 to the end of S2. All time instances were checked manually and erroneous heart cycles were removed to avoid timing errors at this stage.

Each heart cycle was normalized by its maximum amplitude value. The systolic part of the heart cycle, defined as the period ranging from the end of S1 to the beginning of S2, was used in the calculations. Since the discerning information for AS assessment is located in the frequency region above 100 Hz [170], a 5th order Butterworth high-pass filter with a cut-off frequency of 50 Hz was used to emphasize these parts of the signal. The excessive pass-band was chosen to make sure that no valuable information was removed. To reduce the computational complexity, the recorded signals were downsampled to 4.4 kHz. The filtering was performed by zero-phase digital filters, processing the input data in both the forward and reverse directions.

5.1.2 Frequency based features

The large pressure difference across a severely stenotic aortic valve is associated with high frequency murmurs. Conversely, a mild stenosis produces murmurs with lower frequency content [49]. These clinical insights have been formalized in several methods trying to assess the severity of AS using the PCG [49,123,170,223]. Based on joint time-frequency analysis, Donnerstein [49] defined the *dominant frequency* of the murmur as the highest frequency found during systole, see figure 5.3. The time-frequency plane is thresholded at -25 dB of the sound intensity level, a level at which murmurs are no longer considered to be present [223]. Increased AS severity not only causes murmurs to contain a greater portion of higher frequency components, it also prolongs the duration that the ensuing flow produces high frequency murmurs [123]. Another measure of AS severity is consequently the *duration* for which the murmur has a frequency content above a certain threshold frequency, see figure 5.3. According to Tavel et al. [223], the best separation between innocent and pathological murmurs is provided by the duration that the murmur has a frequency content exceeding 200 Hz. In this section, the joint time-frequency analysis was performed by the S-transform, which was defined in section 3.6.1.

A third measure is the *murmur energy ratio* [170] which is defined as the energy between $100 - 500$ Hz (E2) divided by the energy between $20 - 500$ Hz (E1+E2), see figure 5.4 for further details. As the higher frequency content increases with the

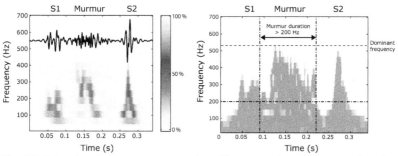

Fig. 5.3: Joint time-frequency representation of heart sounds and a murmur in a dog with mild AS (allocated to subgroup B1). The standard PCG signal is superimposed, showing the first heart sound (S1), the murmur, and the second heart sound (S2). The gray scale represents adjusted (normalized) sound intensity. In the right-hand subplot, the same joint time-frequency representation has been thresholded. The dominant frequency and the duration of systolic frequencies exceeding 200 Hz are marked. Figure based on Höglund et al. [101].

severity of the stenosis, the murmur energy ratio will produce a higher value. In this section, the power spectral density estimate was calculated with Welch's method, see section 3.1. Basically, the murmur energy ratio is similar to measuring the slope of the spectrum. As outlined in chapter 3, this slope is related to the Hurst exponent and thus also to the signal's waveform fractal dimension. Fractal dimensions and other nonlinear measures will be treated more thoroughly in the next section.

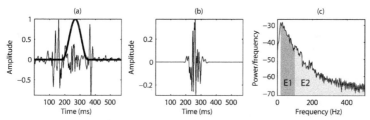

Fig. 5.4: Heart sounds and a murmur in a dog with moderate AS (allocated to subgroup B2 in data set II), together with a window function centered in systole (a). The windowed signal is illustrated in (b). The mean systolic murmur energy is shown in (c), separated into a lower frequency band E1 (20–100 Hz) and a higher frequency band E2 (100–500 Hz). The murmur energy ratio is defined as E2/(E1+E2).

The three frequency based variables were automatically calculated for each heart cycle and averaged over available heart cycles, providing a single mean value per dog. Figure 5.5 presents notched box and whisker plots for the three frequency parameters, plotted as four groups of increasing AS severity (the grouping is defined on page 8). Clearly, there is a trend in all frequency based parameters with higher values for increased AS severity. Using Cuzick's non-parametric test for ordered groups, the significance of this trend can be statistically quantified. There are k groups with sample sizes n_i, $i = 1, 2, \ldots, k$ and a total amount of $N = \sum n_i$ observations. Here, $k = 4$. Each group is given a score l_i according to their relative order. A1, A2, B1 and B2 could be given the scores 1–4, respectively. The outcome from the signal processing algorithms, say the dominant frequency, should then be ranked from 1 to N. The outline of Cuzick's test is then given by equations 5.1–5.5, where L is the weighted sum of the group scores, T is a statistic and R_i is the sum of the ranks in each group. Under the null hypothesis of equal medians, the expected value of T is $E(T)$ and its standard error is given in equation 5.4. The final test statistic is then given by z, which is approximately normally distributed why a corresponding p-value for z may be found in a table over normal distributions with two-tailed areas. Using Cuzick's test, significant trends ($p < 0.05$) were found for the duration above 200 Hz, see table 5.1. Since the murmur energy ratio did not show a significant relation with the ordered groups, this parameter was excluded from further studies. Based on the nonparametric Mann-Whitney U-test with Bonferroni adjustment ($p \leq 0.01$), differences between the subgroups were analyzed in a pairwise manner. The dominant frequency was able to distinguish A2 from B1–B2 and the duration of the murmur above 200 Hz could distinguish between groups B2 and A1–A2.

$$L = \sum_{i=1}^{k} l_i n_i \tag{5.1}$$

$$T = \sum_{i=1}^{k} l_i R_i \tag{5.2}$$

$$E(T) = \frac{1}{2}(N+1)L \tag{5.3}$$

$$\text{std error}(T) = \sqrt{\frac{n+1}{12}\left(N\sum_{i=1}^{k} l_i^2 n_i - L^2\right)} \tag{5.4}$$

$$z = \frac{T - E(T)}{\text{std error}(T)} \tag{5.5}$$

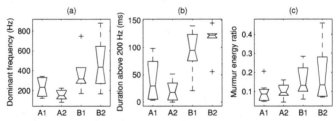

Fig. 5.5: Box and whisker plots with the dominant frequency (a), the duration above 200 Hz (b) and the murmur energy ratio (c) on the y-axes and one box for each group of the murmur on the x-axis. The boxes have lines at the lower quartile, median and upper quartile values, and the notches illustrate the 95% significance level. The whiskers show the extent of the rest of the data and crosses (+) indicate outliers.

It should be noted that AS severity is not a discrete variable but a continuous entity, and dogs with similar obstructions might end up in different groups. For example,

Table 5.1: Regression equations and R-values for all investigated AS assessment algorithms. Also included in the table are p-values obtained from Cuzick's test for ordered groups.

	Parameter	Regression equation	R-value	p-value
1	Dominant frequency	$94.2V_{max} + 40.6$	0.58	0.02
2	Duration (200 Hz)	$22.83e^{0.34V_{max}}$	0.63	0.001
3	Murmur energy ratio	$0.03V_{max} + 0.05$	0.41	0.11
4	Correlation dimension	$1.35\log(1.28V_{max}) + 1.76$	0.69	< 0.001
5	Sample entropy	$0.45\log(0.74V_{max}) + 1.29$	0.70	< 0.001
6	Recurrence rate	$1/(V_{max} + 31.4) - 0.03$	0.56	< 0.001
7	Determinism	$0.004\log(0.6V_{max}) + 0.97$	0.09	0.16
8	Mean diagonal line	$-0.18V_{max} + 36.05$	0.02	0.53
9	Max diagonal line	$-109.5V_{max} + 1802$	0.41	0.07
10	Entropy	$0.03V_{max} + 0.21$	0.42	0.02
11	Laminarity	$-0.01V_{max} + 1.01$	0.36	0.15
12	Trapping time	$1/(V_{max} - 1.29) + 6.97$	0.44	< 0.001
13	Max vertical line	$-4.16V_{max} + 39.9$	0.51	0.001

a dog with a maximum aortic flow velocity of $V_{max} = 3.1$ m/s belongs to group B1 while a dog with $V_{max} = 3.3$ m/s belongs to group B2. It is thus not surprising that the groups are somewhat overlapping. As an alternative to dividing the dogs into groups, the whole material can be investigated as a function of V_{max}. In agreement with the original papers [49, 170], the dominant frequency and the murmur energy ratio were assessed with linear regression (using a first order polynomial) while the duration above 200 Hz was assessed with exponential regression. The obtained R-values were 0.58, 0.63 and 0.41 for the dominant frequency, the murmur duration and the murmur energy ratio, respectively. See table 5.1 for details and figure 5.6 for illustrations of the regression lines.

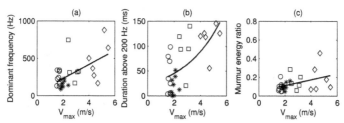

Fig. 5.6: Dominant frequency (a), duration of frequencies above 200 Hz (b) and murmur energy ratio (c) plotted against the aortic flow velocity V_{max} for each dog. The lines illustrate the regression curves calculated for the whole material, and the different markers indicate the four subgroups A1 (∘), A2 (∗), B1 (□) and B2 (◊).

The obtained R-values for the frequency based AS assessment methods are generally lower than what was reported in the original papers [49, 123, 170]. Plausible explanations for these sometimes large differences could be the amount of noise in the data or the differences in canine and human anatomy and etiology. Another reason could be the use of different reference methods, aortic jet velocity compared to transvalvular pressure gradients. However, they both reflect the same physiological phenomenon. Doppler ultrasound measurements of peak aortic flow velocity have also been shown to give excellent correlation with invasive measurements in dogs [133] and are considered appropriate for diagnosis and assessment of AS in humans [29]. In the case of duration of higher frequency components, it is questionable whether the exponential model suggested by Kim et al. [123] is a good choice when applied to the data in this study. Using a first order polynomial gave an R-value of 0.69 compared to 0.63 for the exponential model. Finally, a few modifications were made to the previously defined methods. In the murmur energy ratio, the periodogram was replaced by Welch's power spectral density estimate and in the duration of the high frequency content, the spectrogram was replaced with the S-transform to improve the time resolution. Both these modifications are however improvements compared to the original works.

5.1.3   Nonlinear features

Based on Landau's theory of turbulence [130], fluid flow develops increasing numbers of Fourier modes as the flow velocity increases. At first a few modes dominate, but with stronger forcing the modes become power-law distributed, producing a broad spectrum of eddies at multiple scales. Landau's theory can be used to motivate the spectral measures for AS assessment. As the stenosis become more severe, the flow velocity will increase and so will the amount of Fourier modes. Smaller sized eddies will give rise to higher frequency vibrations, and these are quantified by the spectral based methods mentioned above. An alternative account for the onset of turbulence, the Ruelle-Takens-Newhouse model [200], suggests that turbulence can be described by strange attractors in state space. Strange attractors are commonly characterized by their Lyapunov spectrum, fractal dimension or entropy, and such analysis tools will be investigated in the upcoming sections.

Surrogate data analysis was used to test the adequacy of applying nonlinear techniques. 500 surrogate data sets were created from each murmur data set by randomizing the phases of the original signal's Fourier spectrum [208]. A test statistic for higher order moments [208] was applied and the result from the original data were compared to the result from the surrogate data using a two-tailed Mann-Whitney U-test ($p < 0.05$). This analysis showed that the PCG signals could be assumed nonlinear in 24 out of 27 dogs.

Correlation dimension
It has been suggested that the multiscale structure associated with turbulence in fluids can be described by fractals [149] and that there is a strong interaction between the turbulence and its radiated sound field [241]. It is thus reasonable to assume that the flow behavior causing the murmur can be characterized by the fractal dimension as measured from the PCG signal. Here the correlation dimension D_2, as defined in section 3.4.2, will be used to estimate the fractal dimension. An example obtained from one dog with mild AS is illustrated in figure 5.7, where D_2 was calculated using a time delay $\tau = 3.3$ ms and increasing embedding dimensions ($d = 1 \ldots 15$). There is a clearly defined scaling region ranging from $0.03 - 0.1$ wherein the correlation

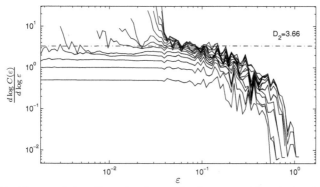

Fig. 5.7: The correlation dimension for one dog from group B1 calculated for embedding dimensions $d = 1, \ldots, 15$. Note the scaling region from $\varepsilon = 0.03 - 0.1$.

dimension can be determined as $D_2 = 3.66$.

Determining the correlation dimension in this way requires some manual meddling before a value of the dimension is obtained. Takens' estimator $T_2(\varepsilon)$, defined in equation 3.51, partially resolves the problem by choosing the scaling range semi-automatically. In this section, $T_2(\varepsilon)$ was calculated using $\varepsilon = 0.13$ as an upper limit of the scaling range, $d = 5$ as the embedding dimension (estimated with Cao's method [38]) and $\tau = 3.3$ ms as the time delay (estimated with auto mutual information [70]). The effect of temporal correlations were reduced by omitting samples that were temporally located less than 1.8 ms apart. The obtained $T_2(\varepsilon)$-value was then used as a measure of AS severity.

All available murmur segments were concatenated into one large set of murmur data for each dog to obtain data sequences of long duration (thereby providing a single value of the signal's fractal dimension per dog). This is important to facilitate the estimation of the correlation sum $C(\varepsilon)$, which requires stationary data of long duration and with high signal to noise ratio. A problem with the correlation dimension measure is that the PCG signal is inherently nonstationary. However, to obtain a "more" stationary signal, only the systolic segments were considered in the analysis. Further, a high pass filter at 50 Hz was applied to remove long range correlations and to emphasize interesting signal properties. It should be noted that high pass filtering the data is similar to bleaching, a processing step that has been advised against when it comes to nonlinear or chaotic data analysis [224].

Figure 5.8 presents a notched box and whisker plot for the correlation dimension as determined by Takens' estimator. Based on the Mann-Whitney U-test with Bonferroni adjustment ($p < 0.01$), significant differences were found between subgroup B2 and A1–A2. As the obstruction becomes more severe, more complex flow conditions will appear, causing a sound signal with higher fractal dimension. The relationship between the correlation dimension and V_{max}, modeled with a logarithmic fit, is presented in figure 5.8. Note that a correlation dimension less than two is usually a contradiction to chaotic flow. In this case, these results are probably due to temporal correlations. The regression line was defined according to table 5.1, and resulted in an R statistic of 0.69. The logarithmic model was chosen in accordance with the turbulence hypothesis. At the onset of turbulence, larger vortices transfer their energy to faster but smaller sized vortices. With increasing flow velocity, ever smaller vortices of ever higher velocities are created until they finally turn into heat by dissipation. The large vortices that are dominant at low flow velocities cause low frequency vibrations that are transmitted to the chest surface. With increasing flow velocities (more severe stenoses), higher frequency vibrations are introduced. These vibrations are also transmitted to the chest surface, but they contain less energy to start with and are further dampened by the tissue. It is thus conceivable that a measure reflecting the amount of turbulence, estimated through the recorded sound signal, will saturate similarly to a logarithmic model.

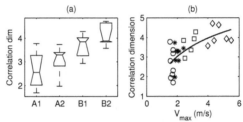

Fig. 5.8: Box and whisker plot with the correlation dimension versus AS severity (a). In (b), the correlation dimension is plotted against the aortic flow velocity V_{max} for each dog. The line illustrates a logarithmic regression curve, $R = 0.69$, as calculated for the whole material. The different markers indicate the four subgroups A1 ($\circ$), A2 ($*$), B1 ($\square$) and B2 ($\diamond$). See figure 5.5 for further explanations.

Among eleven dogs with significant AS (group B), seven dogs had subvalvular lesions and four had valvular changes. Because there was no difference in aortic flow velocity between these dogs, disease severity was considered similar. When comparing the murmur characteristics of the two groups, the correlation dimension was found to be significantly higher in dogs with subvalvular AS. The small sample size should give rise to caution when interpreting these results. However, from a fluid dynamic point of view, subvalvular AS is likely to cause more complex flow patterns than valvular AS. Because subvalvular stenoses are often asymmetric, dynamically changing jets adhere to one or several of the leaflets, causing interactions between the flow and several anatomic structures. If the correlation dimension is able to reflect these differences, it is a very interesting observation. However, a thorough investigation of this finding requires a controlled in vitro investigation, which is out of the scope of this book.

The greatest problems when using chaos based signal analysis tools are that the results are almost always open for interpretation, that nearly noise free data is required and that the amount of data should be large. PCG data is rather cyclostationary than nonstationary, so by concatenating stationary segments, large data sets can be obtained. In this chapter, these segments were simply concatenated in the time domain. A better approach would have been to append the reconstructed state space matrices to each other. An extra flag could then be appended to each coordinate to keep track of the last coordinate in each segment. In this way, false neighbors due to the concatenation procedure could have been excluded from the calculations.

Sample entropy

Estimation of the correlation dimension requires long data sets with very high signal to noise ratio [182]. In fact, convergence of the correlation dimension does not necessarily imply chaos, but may instead be a result of an insufficient amount of data. Sample entropy ($SampEn$) was originally introduced as an unbiased measure of regularity, or complexity, applicable to finite and noisy data sets [198]. Since its introduction, $SampEn$ has successfully been used to classify various biological data such as heart rate variability signals [82, 198] and EEG signals [196]. In the original definition of $SampEn$, see equation 3.62 on page 67, the time delay was set to $\tau = 1$. However, according to dynamical systems theory, this choice is not optimal due to strong time correlations between successive samples. Therefore, a modified version of $SampEn$ [82]) was developed to investigate AS severity. Here auto mutual information was used to determine the time delay compared to the auto correlation function which was used by Govindan et al. [82]. This provides a novel approach to determine $SampEn$.

The embedding dimension was set to $d = 2$ when calculating $SampEn$. This value is too low to unfold the attractor properly, but the limited amount of data does not allow a higher embedding dimension. In fact, Cao's method suggests that an embedding dimension of $d = 5$ is necessary to unfold the attractor properly. It requires a large amount of data to sample such a reconstructed state space dense enough, more data than is available in data set II. To avoid problems (such as false convergence of the correlation dimension and underestimated entropy values) that may arise when the state space is insufficiently covered, a lower embedding dimension was chosen here. Even though $d = 2$ is not enough, such a choice is still useful since entropy measures converge with fewer data points while still being able to quantify changes in system dynamics for lower d-values [232]. Based on the results in this book, it is not possible to claim that the PCG signal stems from a low-dimensional deterministic system or that $SampEn$ represents "true" entropy, but the results do show that $SampEn$ is a parameter able to classify physiological murmurs from murmurs caused by mild AS.

Figure 5.9 presents a notched box and whisker plot for $SampEn$. Based on the Mann-Whitney U-test ($p < 0.01$), significant differences were found between group B1 and A1–A2 and between B2 and A1–A2. The significant difference between subgroup B1 (those with mild AS) and A1–A2 is clinically very interesting. Dogs in group B1 has auscultated murmur grades of II to IV, whereas murmur grades in subgroups A1 and A2 were of either grade I or II. This overlap between the auscultatory results means that in dogs with a grade II murmur, it is not possible to determine the cause of the murmur via auscultation alone [193]. Sample entropy is thus able to distinguish murmurs which are indistinguishable with auscultation.

This result is however based on a small number of dogs, and more data is necessary to draw relevant conclusions.

The relationship between $SampEn$ and V_{max}, modeled with a logarithmic[1] fit, is presented in figure 5.9. The regression line was defined according to table 5.1, and resulted in an R statistic of 0.70.

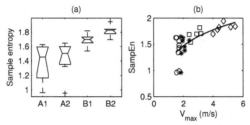

Fig. 5.9: Box and whisker plot with sample entropy versus AS severity (a). In (b), sample entropy is plotted against the aortic flow velocity V_{max} for each dog. The line illustrates a logarithmic regression curve, $R = 0.70$, as calculated for the whole material. The different markers indicate the four subgroups A1 (◦), A2 (∗), B1 (□) and B2 (◇). See figure 5.5 for further explanations. Part of the figure is from Ahlstrom et al. [8].

The same issues that affected the correlation dimension, described in the last section, also apply to $SampEn$. The main difference between the methods is that ε and d are fixed when calculating the correlation sum in $SampEn$. It is important to realize that $SampEn$ is an approximation of entropy which might not coincide with actual entropy. It is however able to distinguish data stemming from different dynamical conditions. When calculating the correlation dimension or when trying to estimate the true entropy of a system, using high pass filters to preprocess the data might not be very suitable. However, when using $SampEn$ to differentiate between different time series, it has been indicated that bleaching the data may improve the classification performance [82].

Nonstationarities in PCG signals arise as an effect of pulsatile blood flow. In the presence of a stenotic aortic valve, the systolic part of the signal becomes increasingly more nonstationary with the severity of the stenosis. Both the amplitude and the amount of higher frequencies increase in mid systole, and as a consequence, the PCG signal becomes more complex. Under the present circumstances, this nonstationarity will actually contribute to $SampEn$ in a favorable manner.

Recurrence quantification analysis
Recurrence plots facilitate visualization of high dimensional spaces, see section 3.6.2. Since recurrence plots can be used on rather short, both linear and nonlinear, nonstationary time series [252], they are appropriate tools for analyzing PCG signals.

In agreement with the original reference [7], the data were downsampled to 14.7 kHz instead of the 4.4 kHz used in the other AS assessment methods presented in

---

[1]A logarithmic fit was chosen for the same reasons as it was chosen in the correlation dimension case.

this chapter. To get quantifiable measures of AS severity, recurrence quantification analysis (RQA) was applied to the systolic period of each heart cycle in each
dog. The obtained RQA values were then averaged for all heart cycles within each
recording, resulting in eight feature values per dog (recurrence rate, determinism,
mean diagonal line length, maximum diagonal line length, entropy, laminarity, trapping time and maximum vertical line length). Four parameters showed significant
relations with the four subgroups according to Cuzick's test ($p < 0.05$), see table
5.1. Of these four features, three showed significant changes between some of the
subgroups according to the Mann-Whitney U-test test after Bonferroni adjustment.
Recurrence rate was significantly different between group A1 and B1–B2 as well as
between A2 and B1–B2, trapping time between group A1 and B1–B2 and between
A2 and B2 and finally maximum vertical line length between A1 and B2. Figure
5.10 provides box and whisker plots for the eight RQA parameters.

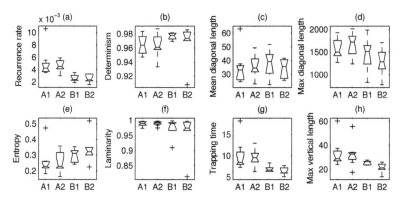

Fig. 5.10: Box and whisker plots of the eight parameters obtained via recurrence quantification analysis versus the severity of AS. See figure 5.5 for further explanations.
Figure from Ahlstrom et al. [7].

The four parameters that showed significant relations with the four subgroups according to Cuzick's test might be interpreted as follows. The recurrence rate corresponds to the probability that a specific state will recur, and as the turbulence
increases, the probability of recurring states decreases. This is in agreement with
figure 5.10a. Entropy reflects the complexity of the deterministic structure in the
system. As the turbulence increases, the complexity of the signal increases, see
figure 5.10e. Trapping time is related with the laminarity time of the system, i.e.
how long the system remains in a specific state. This measure should decrease with
increasing turbulence, as in figure 5.10g. The maximal vertical line length represents
the longest segment which remains in the same phase space region over some time.
This kind of structure in state space will also decrease with increasing turbulence,
in agreement with figure 5.10h.

Most of the RQA features seem to have an on/off property, where physiological
murmurs (group A) are separated from pathological murmurs (group B). Due to this
property, RQA is not a very good tool for assessing the severity of AS. Regression

statistics relating the RQA parameters with aortic flow velocity are nevertheless reported in table 5.1 and in figure 5.11. The clinically interesting task of separating physiological murmurs from pathological murmurs will be further investigated in the next section.

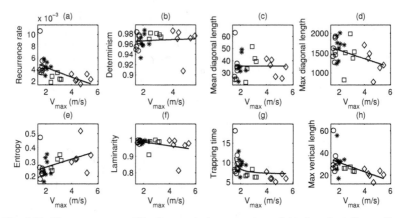

Fig. 5.11: Recurrence quantification analysis parameters plotted against the aortic flow velocity V_{max} for each dog. The lines illustrate the regression curves, see table 5.1 for details. The different markers indicate the four subgroups A1 (○), A2 (∗), B1 (□) and B2 (◇).

5.1.4 Classifying AS from physiological murmurs

The task of differentiating physiological murmurs from murmurs caused by AS can be approached with the same techniques as the AS assessment tools presented in sections 5.1.2–5.1.3. The main difference is that two groups are to be distinguished from each other rather than trying to assign a continuous value as a measure of AS severity. In data set II, group A contains murmurs from physiologically insignificant obstructions while group B contains murmurs recorded from subjects with pathological lesions. Successful separation between the two groups has great clinical significance. By separating physiological murmurs from pathological murmurs, only a certain amount of the patients has to be referred to the cardiology clinic. This would not only save money, but it would also alleviate patients from needless anxiety.

Discrimination abilities of individual features
The probability that the two groups, A and B, comes from distributions with different medians was calculated for each feature by the Mann-Whitney U-test ($p < 0.05$). Results are reported in table 5.2, along with ranges for the feature values separated as group A and group B. Significant differences between the groups, with 95% confidence, were found for all features but the murmur energy ratio, determinism, mean diagonal line length and laminarity. Receiver operating characteristic (ROC) curves

Table 5.2: Range, significance values (Mann-Whitney U-test), area under ROC curve (AUC), sensitivity (%) and specificity (%) for the thirteen parameters when used to distinguish group A from group B in data set II. Results reported as (−) indicates that a negative predictive value of 100% was never achieved.

Parameter	Range (A)	Range (B)	p-value	AUC	Sens	Spec
Dominant frequency (Hz)	85–343	167–878	< 0.001	0.84	100	50
Duration (200 Hz) (ms)	0–98	20–145	< 0.001	0.86	100	44
Murmur energy ratio	0.05–0.21	0.06–0.46	0.09	0.71	100	25
Correlation dimension	1.70–3.78	2.94–4.71	< 0.001	0.93	100	50
Sample entropy	0.96–1.65	1.54–1.95	< 0.001	0.96	100	56
RQA: Recurrence rate	0.003–0.011	0.001–0.003	< 0.001	0.98	100	88
RQA: Determinism	0.933–0.987	0.908–0.986	0.09	0.70	−	−
RQA: Mean diag line	23.0–63.1	22.3–51.7	0.54	0.58	−	−
RQA: Max diag line	1238–2014	776–1988	0.05	0.72	100	6
RQA: Entropy	0.16–0.47	0.23–0.52	0.02	0.78	100	50
RQA: Laminarity	0.973–0.997	0.814–0.998	0.13	0.68	−	−
RQA: Trapping time	6.3–18.1	5.1–8.3	< 0.001	0.93	100	63
RQA: Max vert line	17.4–60.3	13.8–29.6	< 0.001	0.87	100	63

were also calculated for each feature, figure 5.12, and the area under the ROC curve (AUC) is presented in table 5.2.

Since the main application for an AS classification device is screening, the threshold for distinguishing group A from group B was chosen to obtain an optimal negative predictive value. The sensitivity and the specificity of the different features, calculated to give a negative predictive value of 100%, are presented in table 5.2. Based on these results, the best features for classifying AS are the dominant frequency, the duration above 200 Hz, the correlation dimension, the sample entropy, the recurrence rate, entropy, trapping time and the maximum vertical line length. In the next section, combinations of several of these features will be used in the classification process.

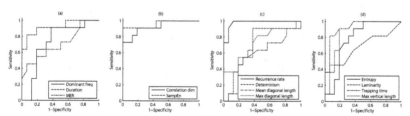

Fig. 5.12: Receiver operating characteristic curves for all features. MER is the murmur energy ratio and Duration is the duration for which the murmur exceeds 200 Hz.

Multi-feature discrimination

A simple ranking of each feature's classification efficiency was obtained based on p-values from Mann-Whitney U-test. Inserting these features in a linear discriminant classifier and evaluating the results with a leave-one-out approach, a feature set with five features (recurrence rate, sample entropy, trapping time, correlation dimension and the duration above 200 Hz) gave the highest amount of correct detections, see figure 5.13. This feature set is, however, far from optimal since some of the features are mutually correlated. A solution to this problem could have been to select the second feature as a weighted sum of its ranking and its correlation with the first feature. Additional features could then have been added in a generalized manner.

The classification rate obtained with an optimal feature set was also investigated, see figure 5.13. The optimal set was found with brute-force, where all possible combinations of features were evaluated. Already with two features, the optimal feature set outperformed the best feature ranking set. With four features, perfect classification results were obtained. However, when more features were added to the feature set, the performance of the classifier started to decrease. The reason is that many different solutions are consistent with the training examples, but disagree on unseen data (overfitting). An example of the optimal three dimensional feature space, constructed with the parameters sample entropy, duration above 200 Hz and recurrence rate, is illustrated in figure 5.14. This section have highlighted the importance of proper features and appropriate feature selection.

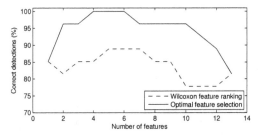

Fig. 5.13: The percentage of correct detections as a function of the number of features used to classify physiological murmurs from murmurs caused by aortic stenosis.

5.1.5   Additional comments

The results obtained in this section on AS assessment were derived using all available data in data set II, and should be cross validated accordingly. Another limitation is that subjects with significant AS and left-sided congestive heart failure have a diminished and sometimes undetectable murmur. This important patient group is not represented in the data used for this study. Both these issues are currently under investigation by our research group, where a larger data set recorded from human patients is to be used.

All presented variables are invariant features of the murmur signal. However, murmurs stem from turbulent blood flow, which varies in time as a result of the pulsatile flow. Tracking changes in various properties such as maximum and mean frequency over time would provide additional information about the characteristic features

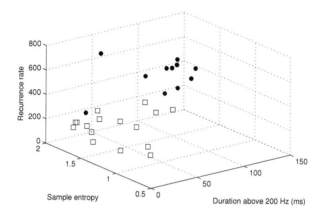

Fig. 5.14: Example of a three dimensional feature space spanned by the duration above 200 Hz, SampEn and recurrence rate. The squares represent group A and the circles represent group B.

and the underlying dynamics of the murmur. Such time-variable properties would probably be better suited for detecting subtle pathologic changes in anatomic structures; however, such time-variable features would be considerably more complicated to interpret, both for the physician and in an automated computer analysis.

It should be noted that the requirements on a PCG classification system differ depending on the age group or population under investigation. For example, different age groups lead to the following scenarios:

1. *Screening in a young population.* Physiological murmurs are very common in children, and a method able to separate physiological murmurs from pathological murmurs would be of great value. However, the performance requirements are extremely high. For example, a physiological murmur has to be separated from a very mild murmur caused by AS due to the latter's implications on choice of profession, insurance issues and whether follow-ups of a possible disease are needed or not. Due to the consequences of an incorrect diagnosis, the tolerance for false positives and negatives is low and the performance requirements on the system are huge.

2. *Measuring the degree of stenosis in the elderly.* Pathological changes in the aortic valves are common in the elderly. Usually this change has little physiological importance when the stenosis is mild. However, it is important to find those patients who really have a significant narrowing of the valve opening since surgical correction may improve the prognosis considerably. The classification task is then to measure the degree of the stenosis and decide whether the stenosis is mild or moderate to severe. This scenario is easier so solve since the grey area between a physiological murmur and a mild stenosis is out of interest.

5.2   Assessing and classifying regurgitant systolic murmurs

Regurgitant flow through the mitral or tricuspid valves causes a murmur that typically begins with atrioventricular valve closure and continues till semilunar valve closure. Because the pressure gradient between ventricle and atrium is large throughout systole, the murmur tends to have a constant intensity throughout systole (holosystolic). The appearance of a murmur caused by an insufficient mitral valve is illustrated in figure 5.15.

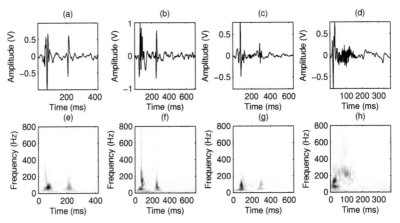

Fig. 5.15: PCG signals with different degrees of mitral insufficiency (normal (N), mild MI (M1), moderate MI (M2) and severe MI (M3) in (a)–(d), respectively). Corresponding joint time-frequency representations are illustrated in (e)–(h).

The mitral valve apparatus consists of five different structures; mitral annulus, leaflets, chordae tendineae, papillary muscles and the free wall of the left ventricle. Malfunction in any of these may result in MI. Murmurs caused by MI begin with systole and continues as long as the left ventricular pressure exceeds that of the enlarged left atrium. The murmur often engulfs the aortic component of S2 but stops before the pulmonary component. In acute MI the murmur might even be diamond-shaped, loud (grade IV or more) and does not necessarily extend to the end of systole. Since the valve closure is incomplete, blood is leaving the ventricle through both the aorta and the left atrium. This causes a decrease in the rate of rise of the ventricular pressure which weakens the intensity of S1. The presence of an S3 suggests that the incompetence is significant, although it does not necessarily imply systolic dysfunction or elevated filling pressure as it usually does.

In tricuspid insufficiency, the holosystolic murmur increases with inspiration. Unlike MI the murmur of tricuspid insufficiency engulfs the pulmonary component of S2. In mild cases, S4 may be present.

142

The remainder of this section, which is based on results from Ljungvall et al. [141], will deal with signal analysis methods attempting to assess MI severity. The 77 dogs from data set III, see page 9 for details, will be used in the evaluation. The outline of this section deviates somewhat from Ljungvall et al. [141] as only the echocardiographic findings are used as a reference for disease severity (auscultation results were also used as a reference in [141]). The dogs were classified as normal (N) if no signs of anatomical- or functional cardiac pathology could be found. Estimation of MI severity was based on the obtained echocardiographic information into mild (M1), moderate (M2) and severe (M3). Another difference is that only the LA/Ao-ratio was used as a reference in Ljungvall et al. [141] while also the LVID-parameters are included here.

It has been shown that the progression of mitral regurgitation is associated with certain characteristic changes in the PCG signal. The murmur increases in duration from early or late systolic to holosystolic, the amplitude of the murmur increases, the duration of systole decreases regardless of heart rate, and there is a shift in the amplitude ratio between S1 and S2 [99, 129, 226]. The use of signal analysis techniques for investigating MI have mainly focused on classification between physiological and pathological murmurs [213] and on classification between different cardiac abnormalities [113, 142, 235]. Ljungvall et al. [141] provides the first attempt to assess MI severity based on signal analysis of PCG signals. The features to be investigated are listed below.

1. Energy in S1.
2. Energy in S2.
3. Duration for which the murmur exceeds 200 Hz.
4. First frequency peak.
5. Murmur energy ratio.
6. Sample entropy.
7. Auto mutual information.

5.2.1 Pre-processing

Aided by the ECG recording, all recorded PCG signals will be manually segmented. Four markers per heart cycle are determined; the beginning of the first heart sound, the end of the first heart sound, the beginning of the second heart sound and the end of the second heart sound. Noisy or corrupted signal segments, determined by visual inspection, will be excluded from further studies. To reduce computational complexity and to remove high frequency noise, the data will also be downsampled to 4.4 kHz. A 5th order zero-phase Butterworth high-pass filter with a cut-off frequency of 30 Hz emphasizes the discerning information in the PCG signal and reduces low-frequency noise.

5.2.2 Features

The seven measures listed above will automatically be derived and their abilities to assess MI severity will be investgated. Many of these features are similar to the ones used for AS assessment, and the descriptions will consequently be rather concise in this section.

In dogs, it is generally believed that S1 becomes louder while S2 decreases in intensity with increasing MI severity [129]. To account for these changes, the energy of the segments containing S1 and S2 can be investigated. Unfortunately, each recording will depend on chest size, skin thickness and the interface between the skin and the stethoscope. Direct comparison of sound intensity or energy is thus impossible. To circumvent this problem, the energy in S1 and S2 can be normalized against the energy in diastole. Using diastole to estimate the noise level in PCG signals has previously been employed by Durand et al. [53], and since the dogs in data set III are all free from diastolic murmurs, this seems to be a feasible approach. The energy in both S1 and S2 can be calculated as the normalized energy within the S1 and S2 segments. These two values will be determined in each heart cycle and averaged across available heart cycles. From the boxplots in figure 5.16, it is obvious that the energy in S2 decreases with increasing MI severity. According to Cuzick's non-parametric trend test for ordered groups, it can be shown that this trend is significant ($p < 0.001$). This also agrees with intuition (S2 decreases in intensity as forward stroke volume is reduced) as well as with previous results [99]. More interestingly, there are no trends that S1 should increase in energy. This is an interesting result since it contradicts current beliefs when it comes to dogs. However, the understanding that S1 should increase in intensity is mostly based on auscultatory findings [81]. Perhaps S1 merely sounds louder as an effect of decreased S2 intensity in combination with a vigorous murmur. After all, the prevailing opinion in humans is that S1 decreases in intensity with increasing MI severity [226]. Looking at the trend in figure 5.16, this also seems to be the case in dogs. In contrast to the trend in S2, the decrease in S1 in not statistically significant ($p = 0.14$). In fact, according to Cuzick's trend test, the energy in S1 is the only feature in this study which does not show a significant trend in relation to MI severity.

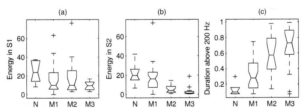

Fig. 5.16: Box and whisker plots with the energy in S1 (a), the energy in S2 (b) and duration of frequencies exceeding 200 Hz (c) on the y-axes and one box for each group of the murmur on the x-axis. The boxes have lines at the lower quartile, median and upper quartile values, and the notches illustrate the 95% significance level. The whiskers show the extent of the rest of the data and crosses (+) indicate outliers.

The duration for which a murmur is present in systole changes with the severity of MI as the murmur shifts from early or late systolic to holosystolic [161]. Since even a small regurgitant jet causes rather loud murmurs with high frequency content, this duration can readily be measured as the percentage of systole where the murmur has a frequency content exceeding 200 Hz. This particular feature was introduced by Kim et al. [123] for assessing AS severity, and an illustration describing the feature extraction methodology was shown in figure 5.3. As before, the duration can be measured in each cardiac cycle and averaged across available heart cycles. In the boxplot in figure 5.16, it can be seen that the duration for which the systolic frequency content exceeds 200 Hz is nearly nonexisting in normal dogs. Mild MI is characterized by an early or late systolic murmur of short duration while moderate and severe MI are associated with a holosystolic murmur of long duration.

The first frequency peak is a measure of the murmur's harshness [61]. This peak can be estimated via Welch's spectral estimate or any other non-parametric spectral estimation technique. However, a more accurate power spectrum can be obtained with a parametric model, especially when the signal is of short duration [217]. Here, a 4th order AR model is used (see section 3.1 for details on AR models). AR models are good at representing peaks in the frequency spectrum. According to Akaike's information criterion[2], this model order is slightly too small. However, it is deliberately chosen on the small side to avoid spurious low-frequency peaks. The poles corresponding to the AR coefficients determine where the peaks in the estimated power spectrum will be located. The first frequency peak belongs to the pole with the smallest angle, and can be determined as the minimum angle of the complex roots of the AR polynomials. An example is shown in figure 5.17. Here the AR model was constructed by concatenating all systolic segments within each recording, and one frequency peak value was determined per dog based on this batch of data. Figure 5.18 indicates that the frequency spectrum is shifted towards higher frequencies with increasing MI severity, a result that agrees with previous work [162].

The murmur energy ratio, see figure 5.4, quantifies the amount of higher frequencies in the murmur [170]. Here a periodogram was calculated for each systolic segment, where every segment was zero-padded to get the same length. Available periodograms where then averaged to get a final spectral estimate per dog (note the resemblance to Welch's method). The murmur energy ratio was defined as the energy between 50-500 Hz divided by the energy between 20-500 Hz. With increasing severity of valvular lesions, the larger retrograde volume and the decreased average regurgitant velocity produce a murmur with a "harsher" quality. A hypothesis for this phenomenon was put forward by Tavel [222], suggesting that the increased harshness originates as an effect of much lower frequency contributions. From figure 5.18, the murmur energy ratio increases with increasing MI severity. This indicates that it is more likely an intensification of medium frequency components that causes the altered sound.

---

[2]Akaike's information criterion is often used to estimate the model order [217]. It is defined as $AIC(m) = N \ln(\sigma_p^2) + 2m$, where N is the length of the signal, σ_p^2 is the prediction error and m is the model order. The model order is set to the m that minimizes $AIC(m)$.

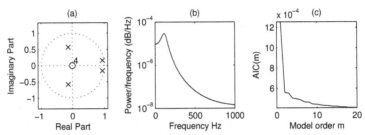

Fig. 5.17: Pole/zero plot with complex conjugated poles corresponding to the roots of the AR polynomials (a). The minimum angle to the roots determines the first frequency peak, which is shown in (b) after scaling with the sample frequency (only a portion of the spectral estimate is shown). Akaike's information criterion, AIC(m), indicates a model order higher than the one used, m=4 (c).

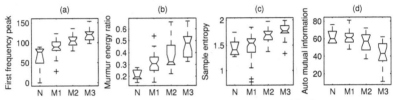

Fig. 5.18: Box and whisker plots with the first frequency peak (a), the murmur energy ratio (b), the sample entropy (c) and the auto mutual information (d) on the y-axes and one box for each group of the murmur on the x-axis. For other explanations see figure 5.16.

Two nonlinear parameters will also be investigated. Sample entropy and rate of decrease of the auto mutual information function. Sample entropy will be derived according to section 3.4.4, using sequences of length $d = 2$ and a tolerance level of $\varepsilon = 0.2\sigma$, where σ is the standard deviation of the murmur signal. Results from figure 5.18 show that sample entropy increases with increasing MI severity. This can be explained by a more complex flow behavior that gives rise to more irregular murmurs. The auto mutual information (AMI) represents the mean predictability of future samples based on previous samples, and is often considered a nonlinear analogue to the autocorrelation function [70], see section 3.4. A complicated signal is less predictable compared to a straightforward signal, so the rate of decrease of the AMI function will depend on the complexity of the signal [188]. Both sample entropy and AMI attempts to estimate the complexity of a signal, but where sample entropy is a statistic that quantifies the regularity in the time series, AMI tries to detect nonlinear dependencies. Further, the AMI function is able to investigate time scale dependence through τ [105]. Here the first local minimum of the AMI function was used as a measure of the rate of decrease. Since the mean predictability decreases with increasing signal complexity, the results from the AMI analysis (figure 5.18) show lower values for more severe MI. Since both nonlinear measures perform better with long time series, all systolic segments within each recording were concatenated and one feature value per dog was determined based on this batch of data.

5.2.3 MI assessment

In section 5.1, all PCG-derived variables were fit to the maximum aortic flow velocity by regression models. This was a suitable approach since the flow velocity correlates very well with AS severity. In MI assessment, the situation is more complicated since there is no single parameter able to fully characterize the integrity of the mitral valve [255]. To be able to investigate how the dependent variable (extracted from the PCG signal) is affected by many different independent variables (such as echocardiographic parameters), the usual regression model has to be generalized. To investigate relations between several variables, a multiple regression model can be used [27]. This model is defined in equation 5.6. The dependent variable Y is, possibly, affected by the independent variables $X_1, X_2, \ldots, X_k$ when combined using a set of regression parameters $\alpha_1, \alpha_2, \ldots, \alpha_k$ plus a constant α_0. The values of Y are also affected by a random variable e, which is assumed to be normally distributed with zero mean.

$$Y = \alpha_0 + \alpha_1 X_1 + \alpha_2 X_2 + \ldots + \alpha_k X_k + e \tag{5.6}$$

Using gender, age, breed, body weight, heart rate and echocardiographic variables (La/Ao-ratio, FS, percent increase in LVIDd and LVIDs above expected values) as independent variables, multiple regression equations for each of the extracted sound features can be calculated, see table 5.3. The adjusted R^2, see table 5.3, represents the amount of variation in the dependent variable that the model is able to account for. Adjusted basically means that the usual R^2 value has been modified to account for the number of independent variables in the model and for the number of independent variables that the model is based upon. In table 5.3, the sound variables seem to either correlate with an increase in LVIDd$_{inc}$ accompanied with a decrease in LVIDs$_{inc}$ or with the La/Ao-ratio. This is actually not the case but rather an effect of collinearity between the variables. Since there is an obvious correlation between different measures of MI severity, only the best results are reported here.

When constructing a descriptive model, only a subset of the independent variables is likely to be needed. A few basic approaches, similar to the feature selection approaches introduced in section 3.10, are:

- *Forward selection:* The independent variable that explains most of the variations in the dependent variable is chosen first. The second variable is chosen as the one that, together with the first, best describes variations in the dependent variable. This process is continued until additional variables do not significantly increase the accuracy of the model.

- *Backward selection:* Start with all the independent variables and remove the least significant variables one at a time until only significant variables remain.

- *Stepwise selection:* Perform a forward selection, but remove variables which are no longer significant after the introduction of new variables.

Here, the multiple regression analysis was performed in a backward stepwise manner by starting with all variables included in the model and then step-wise removing the variable with the highest p-value until all the remaining variables had a p-value

Table 5.3: Summary of prediction formulas obtained from multiple regression analysis when relating the sound features to the echocardiographic and signalment variables.

Parameter	Prediction formula	R^2-value	p-value
Energy in S1	$26.2 - 7.5 \cdot \text{La/Ao}$	0.04	0.05
Energy in S2	$32.7 - 14.1 \cdot \text{La/Ao}$	0.24	< 0.001
Duration above 200 Hz	$0.4 + 0.01 \cdot \text{LVIDd}_{inc} - 0.01 \cdot \text{LVIDs}_{inc}$	0.46	< 0.001
First frequency peak	$70.7 - 0.24 \cdot \text{HR} + 36.7 \cdot \text{La/Ao}$	0.40	< 0.001
Murmur energy ratio	$0.1 + 0.2 \cdot \text{La/Ao}$	0.34	< 0.001
Sample entropy	$1.6 + 0.01 \cdot \text{LVIDd}_{inc} - 0.01 \cdot \text{LVIDs}_{inc}$	0.24	< 0.001
Auto mutual information	$83.1 - 18.2 \cdot \text{La/Ao}$	0.36	< 0.001

Table 5.4: Summary of prediction formulas obtained from multiple regression analysis when relating the echocardiographic and signalment variables to the sound features.

Parameter	Prediction formula	R^2-value	p-value
La/Ao-ratio	$1.17 + 0.39 \cdot \text{Sample entropy} - 0.0084 \cdot \text{Mutual information} -$ $0.011 \cdot \text{Energy in S2} + 0.84 \cdot \text{Murmur energy ratio}$	0.53	< 0.001
LVIDd$_{inc}$	$-35.4 + 16.9 \cdot \text{Sample entropy} + 0.29 \cdot \text{First frequency peak} -$ $0.47 \cdot \text{Energy in S2}$	0.39	< 0.001
LVIDs$_{inc}$	No model obtained	–	–
FS	$24.8 + 14.2 \cdot \text{Peak frequency} + 15.6 \cdot \text{Murmur energy ratio}$	0.44	< 0.001
HR	$199 - 0.82 \cdot \text{Mutual information} - 0.36 \cdot \text{First frequency peak}$	0.08	0.02

< 0.05. An interesting result is that the PCG-derived features showed an absence of effect in all the included signalment variables (age, gender, breed and body weight).

A limitation with multiple regression is that only linear relationships between the dependent and independent variables are investigated. For example, when plotting the sample entropy against the La/Ao-ratio, it looks as though a logarithmic regression would be more suitable. For other parameters such as the energy in S2, an exponentially declining regression curve seems preferable. In this book, nonlinear relations between variables will however not be investigated.

In table 5.4, the multiple regression was performed the other way around. The results are more or less the same as the ones in table 5.3, but this representation reveals the importance of the results in a better way. For example, variability in the La/Ao-ratio is successfully modeled by an increase in sample entropy, a decrease in auto mutual information, a decrease in the energy in S2 and an increase in the murmur energy ratio. It is very encouraging that these four sound variables correlate well with the La/Ao-ratio – the echocardiographic parameter that, if any, has been found to reliably indicate MI severity in dogs [32].

5.2.4   Distinguishing severe MI

In a veterinary setting, the classification task at hand is to find dogs with severe MI. The reason why this distinction is interesting is that affected dogs progress from mild to severe MI over a rather long period of time, but demonstrate no outward

Table 5.5: Range, significance values (Mann-Whitney U-test), area under ROC curve values (AUC), sensitivity (%) and specificity (%) for the seven parameters when used to distinguish dogs with severe MI.

Parameter	Range (A)	Range (B)	p-value	AUC	Sens	Spec
Energy in S1	0–76	3–17	0.20	0.53	29	78
Energy in S2	0–74	1–19	< 0.001	0.88	82	87
Duration above 200 Hz	0.07–0.98	0.07–0.99	< 0.001	0.78	83	73
First frequency peak	0–135	98–153	< 0.001	0.88	88	82
Murmur energy ratio	0.15–0.66	0.32–0.67	< 0.001	0.86	94	68
Sample entropy	0.77–1.97	1.33–1.99	< 0.001	0.82	76	83
Auto mutual information	37–81	11–62	< 0.001	0.87	71	88

clinical signs until the regurgitant valves cause heart failure in the last stages of the disease. When this happens, heart failure therapy is needed. Following the methodology used in the AS assessment setting (section 5.1), the Mann-Whitney U-test showed excellent separability qualities for most features. In fact, only the energy in S1 had a p-value exceeding 0.001, see table 5.5. The corresponding ROC curves (figure 5.19) also indicate that most individual features had excellent classification performance. For example, the first frequency peak reached a sensitivity of 88%, a specificity of 82% and an AUC of 0.88. These results are, however, derived without cross validation.

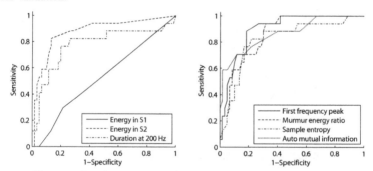

Fig. 5.19: Receiver operating characteristic curves for all features.

Cross validated results, obtained when combining several features in a leave-one-out LDA classification scheme, showed similar performance as the unvalidated first frequency peak (sensitivity=88%, specificity=82% and AUC=0.89). An exhaustive search showed that the smallest feature set with the largest possible amount of correct detections consisted of the first frequency peak, the energy in S2 and the first minimum in the AMI function. For comparison, auscultation performed by experienced veterinarians gave a sensitivity of 70% and a specificity of 97%.

As a complement to this regression-based statistical investigation, it is possible to test differences based on the four ordered MI severity groups. Such analyses were performed in Ljungvall et al. [141], but these details are left out from this section.

Table 5.6: Results from Cuzick's non-parametric trend test for ordered groups (p-value) and the statistically different subgroups as determined with the Mann-Whitney U-test with Bonferroni adjustment.

Parameter	p-value	Significantly different groups
Energy in S1	0.14	–
Energy in S2	< 0.001	M3↔N, M1, M2 and M2↔N, M1
Duration above 200 Hz	< 0.001	N↔M2, M3 and M1↔M2,M3
First frequency peak	< 0.001	M3↔N, M1, M2 and M2↔N, M1
Murmur energy ratio	< 0.001	M3↔N, M1, M2 and N↔M2
Sample entropy	< 0.001	M1↔M2, M3
Auto mutual information	< 0.001	M3↔N, M1, M2

A table summarizing the results can be found in table 5.6. The reason for such an analysis is of course the absence of a single continuous parameter able to describe MI severity. By manually investigating the dogs, all possible data as well as the vast experience of the sonographer is incorporated in the final grouping.

5.2.5 Additional comments

The classification task in this section aimed at distinguishing dogs with severe MI from the other dogs included in the data set. In humans, the situation is somewhat different since correction of MI should be performed well before left ventricular decompensation sets in [30]. A classification system intended for human patients would definitely not be designed to only find severe MI but to also detect moderate MI. The reason for not including mild MI in the pathologic group is that basically all humans have a small but insignificant leakage through the mitral valve. Adjusting the test to be more suitable for human applications, i.e. classification of dogs which are normal or have mild MI from dogs with moderate to severe MI, a correct detection rate of 88% was achieved.

5.3 Classifying murmurs of different origin

The task of classifying murmurs of different origin calls for modified features as well as more advanced classification approaches. Up till now, the severity of the disease could more or less be estimated with a single feature. For example, sample entropy could be used to grade the complexity of the signal and the complexity of the sound signal could be linked to disease severity.

Several authors have investigated the possibility to automatically classify cardiac murmurs. This section will present a survey based on Ahlstrom et al. [11]. The survey covers most features from the literature, ranging from time domain characteristics [39,46,178,210], spectral characteristics [47,211,235], frequency representations with time resolution [46,86,113,135,137,142,229,235] as well as nonlinear and chaos based features [11].

Table 5.7: Summary of all features. Column one through three represents the feature names, the number of features and a short description of the extraction technique, respectively. The stars indicate features not previously used for heart murmur classification.

Shannon energy	9	Envelope values derived from the normalized Shannon energy.
WT entropy	11*	The Shannon entropy of each wavelet (WT) detail and the wavelet approximation using a level 10 decomposition with the Daubechies 2 wavelet.
WT detail	9	The 6th wavelet detail of a level 10 Daubechies 2 wavelet discretized into 9 bins.
ST map	16	Joint time-frequency representation (calculated with the S-transform) in the frequency range 0–150 Hz discretized into a 4x4-matrix.
Eigenvalue	8*	The eight first eigenvalues to the joint time-frequency matrix.
Eigentimes and eigenfrequencies	40*	Two left eigenvectors and two right eigenvectors transformed into distribution functions whose histograms (10 bins) are used as features.
Bispectrum	16*	First non-redundant region of the bispectrum (frequency range 0-300 Hz) discretized into 16 equally sized triangles.
GMM cycle	40*	Gaussian mixture Model (GMM) of the reconstructed state space of the systolic period (including HS).
GMMx murmur	40*	GMM of the reconstructed state space of the systolic period (excluding HS).
VFD	8*	Variance fractal dimension (VFD) values.
RQA	10*	Recurrence Quantification Analysis (RQA).

Compared to previous sections in this chapter, time dependent features will be incorporated in the analysis. This is important in order to be able to pick up the differences between crescendo-decrescendo murmurs and holosystolic murmurs. A great number of features will be extracted and a feature selection algorithm will be employed to determine which features are most useful. The derived feature set will also be used in a neural network classifier to assess its discriminative qualities. The evaluation will be based on data set IV, consisting of 36 patients with AS, MI or physiological murmurs.

5.3.1 Features

A preprocessing step was used before deriving the different features. ECG-gated Shannon energy was used to segment the PCG signals according to chapter 4. The segmentation result was visually inspected and erroneously segmented heart cycles were excluded from the study. Uncertain cases were rather rejected than kept to avoid timing errors when creating the features. The feature extraction process extracted 207 scalar values per heart cycle, and each of these was averaged across available heart cycles. All features were also normalized to zero mean and unit standard deviation. A summary of the different features is given in table 5.7.

Time and frequency based properties

It is generally known that systolic ejection murmurs like AS are crescendo-decrescendo shaped while regurgitant systolic murmurs, like MI, are holosystolic or band-shaped. However, this is not always obvious when looking at actual recorded signals. Using normalized Shannon energy as a measure of intensity, the shape of physiological murmurs (PM) and murmurs caused by AS or MI are shown in figure 5.20. The classical shapes are indicated, but having the standard deviation in mind, the difference in shape is not evident. In the AS and MI cases, the large standard deviations are partly due to the severity of the disease, which is ranging from mild to severe in data set IV. The nine presented instants were selected at times before S1, peak S1, after S1, $1/4$ into systole, $1/2$ into systole, $3/4$ into systole, before S2, peak S2 and finally after S2. The features were derived as mean values of each heart cycle in one patient.

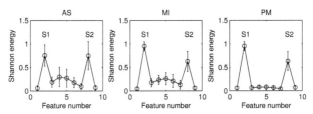

Fig. 5.20: **Mean value of the Shannon energy calculated at nine time instants in systole, the whiskers show the standard deviation.**

Looking at the mean and standard deviation joint time-frequency representations of all available AS, MI and PM cases, figure 5.21, distinct areas can be found in the standard deviation plots. From the figure, it is obvious that there is great variability between different patients within the same group. This is unfortunate when the aim is to classify patients into different categories – ideally all patients with the same disease would behave similarly. Focusing on differences between diseases, it can be seen that the murmur do not change much over systole. The murmur in AS on the other hand seems very unstable. Since the murmur in AS is crescendo-decrescendo shaped, and the peak depends on the severity of the stenosis, it makes sense that the mean of several AS murmurs deviates between patients. Finally, PM are known to be of low frequency, which is verified by the figure.

Joint time-frequency representations are valuable tools when visually inspecting signals, but the amount of information is immense. In a classification setting it is necessary to find a compact representation consisting of a manageable number of features. This issue has been solved in different ways. Gupta et al. [86] and Ölmez et al. [142] chose to only consider one wavelet scale (the second wavelet detail corresponding to 1120 Hz) and discretize it into 32 bins (the actual features are the sum of the absolute values within each bin). Turkoglu et al. [229] used the entropy of each detail and approximation in a complete wavelet packet decomposition and Leung et al. [135] discretized the whole time-frequency matrix (the frequency content was limited to 0–62 Hz) to a 4x4 matrix by downsampling.

Some adaptations were necessary to adjust all of these feature extraction methods

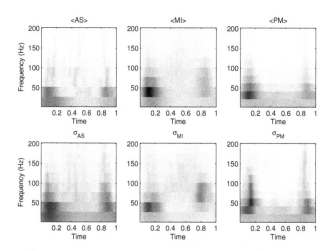

Fig. 5.21: Mean (top) and standard deviation (bottom) time-frequency representations (calculated with the S-transform) of aortic stenosis, mitral insufficiency and physiological murmurs. The time scale was resampled to 2048 samples after calculating the S-transform, and is here represented in arbitrary normalized units.

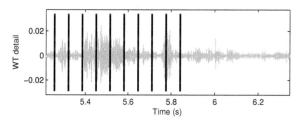

Fig. 5.22: The 6th wavelet detail of one heart cycle from a patient with aortic stenosis. The vertical lines are time markers equidistantly distributed over the region of interest. The absolute sum between each marker constitutes the feature values. Figure from Ahlstrom et al. [11].

to data set IV. Daubechies second wavelet was used due to its similarity with S1 and S2, and a level 10 decomposition of the signal was performed. The systolic part of the 6th level detail was divided into 9 bins, see figure 5.22. The wavelet entropy was calculated for each decomposition (10 details and 1 approximation), not for every wavelet packet as in the work by Turkoglu et al. [229]. Finally, the S-transform was used to calculate the time-frequency matrix which was divided into a 4x4-matrix, see figure 5.23. However, a more generous frequency range was used, 0–150 Hz compared to 0–62 Hz as used by Leung et al. [135].

A different way to represent a time-frequency matrix in a compact manner is to use singular value decomposition. Marinovic and Eichmann [151] simply extracted

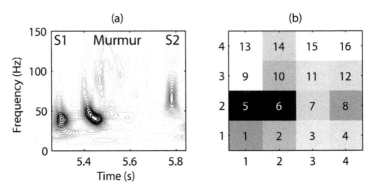

Fig. 5.23: Time-frequency representation (calculated with the S-transform) of one heart cycle from a patient with aortic stenosis (a), S1 can be seen at 5.3s and S2 at 5.8s. In (b) the same data has been discretized into a 4x4 map of features.

the eigenvalues of the time-frequency matrix, and Hassanpour et al. [96] extended the method to also incorporate information from the eigenvectors in an attempt to classify EEG seizures. More specifically, the time-frequency matrix S is decomposed according to $S = Q_1 D Q_2^T$. Q_1 and Q_2 are called the left and the right eigenvectors, or in this particular case eigentime and eigenfrequency, respectively. Here, eigentimes and eigenfrequencies corresponding to the two largest eigenvalues were used to derive the features. Since eigenvectors are orthonormal, the cumulative sum of their squared elements can be considered as density functions. These density functions are nondecreasing, and as can be seen in figures 5.24(d, g, j, m), they have no significant changes in some areas. This can be quantified with histograms, see figures 5.24(e, h, k, n), where only a few of the bins have significant values. The final features are thus constituted by these histograms. In the singular value decomposition calculations, the time-frequency matrix was derived using the S-transform. These features can be interpreted as the main components of the time-frequency matrix. For example, the minima of the first eigentime in figure 5.24(i) correspond to S1, S2 and the murmur.

Higher order statistics

Since methods based on second-order statistics do not take nonlinearity and non-Gaussianity into account, higher order statistics might provide more useful information about the PCG signal. Bispectra for signals from various systolic murmurs are presented in figure 5.25. First of all it can be seen that the bispectra are nonzero, as it would be if the signals were Gaussian. Secondly, the bispectra are not constant, as they would be for linear data. Thirdly, the main frequency content is well below 300 Hz and exhibits distinct peaks. Forth, considerable phase coupling exists between different frequencies. Finally it is also seen that the patterns revealed in the bispectra differ between various pathologies. It has previously been indicated that PCG signals are non-Gaussian [91, 160], but it has not been explicitly stated that this is the case. When performing Hinich's Gaussianity test on each heart cycle in data set IV, it turns out that each and every one of the 445 heart cycles have

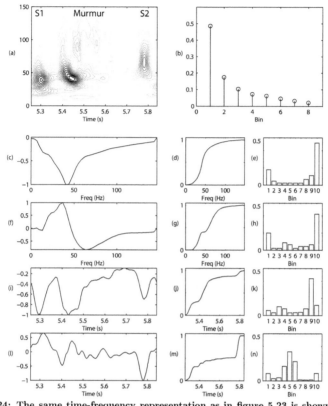

Fig. 5.24: The same time-frequency representation as in figure 5.23 is shown in (a) and its first eight eigenvalues are shown in (b). (c) and (f) illustrate the first and second left eigenvectors, respectively. To the right of the respective figures are their probability distributions, (d, g), and their histograms (e, h). (i-n) are corresponding plots for the first and second right eigenvectors.

zero skewness with probability $p < 0.05$. This strongly suggests that the data are non-Gaussian (nonzero skewness) and that higher-order statistics of PCG signals will reveal new information compared to Fourier analysis. Similarly, a hypothesis regarding linearity could be rejected using Hinich's linearity test (for a nonlinear process, an estimated statistic may be expected to be much larger than a theoretical statistic, and in this case the estimated value is, on average, 3.4 times larger). This motivates the use of the nonlinear techniques in the two upcoming sections.

The bispectrum can be discretized to make the number of quantifying units more manageable [244], see figure 5.26. Due to symmetry, it is enough to investigate the first nonredundant region [167]. Box and whisker plots for the bispectral features are presented in figure 5.27. Unfortunately the features overlap and are more or less useless for classification purposes (the Mann-Whitney U-test shows significant

155

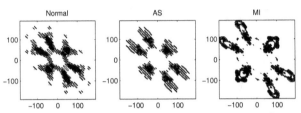

Fig. 5.25: Examples of bispectra from one heart cycle in a normal person, from a patient with aortic stenosis and from a patient with mitral insufficiency. One heart cycle here roughly starts with S1 and ends after S2. All axes represent frequency in Hz.

differences ($p < 0.05$) for feature 2 between AS↔PM, feature 3 between AS↔MI and AS↔PM and feature 7–8 and 11 between MI↔PM). The bispectrum is however still a useful tool and figure 5.25 does reveal a lot of information. There are distinct differences between the various heart valve diseases in figure 5.25, but these differences are clearly lost in the discretization. A different approach is thus needed to extract this information. A few ideas are Gaussian mixture models or perhaps some parametric models like the non-Gaussian AR model, but these issues are left for future studies. If nothing more, the bispectrum can be used as a visualization technique to support the physician's decision.

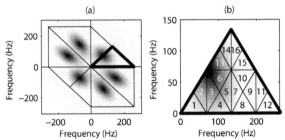

Fig. 5.26: Example of a bispectrum from a patient with aortic stenosis. The different regions of the bispectrum are plotted in (a) where the bold triangle shows the first non-redundant region. In (b) the region of interest is highlighted. The smaller triangles indicate 16 features obtained from the bispectrum, where each feature is calculated as the mean intensity of each triangle. Figure from Ahlstrom et al. [11].

Waveform fractal dimensions

Considering the mere waveform of bioacoustic time series, it appears that these signals possess valid characteristics for pursuing fractal dimension calculations:

- The signals do not self-cross.

- The waveform is often self-affine, i.e. in order to scale the signal, a different scaling factor is required for each axis. In physical systems, this property is not strict but probabilistic, and there are minimum and maximum scaling limits (depending on the accuracy of the measurement, the sampling resolution etc.).

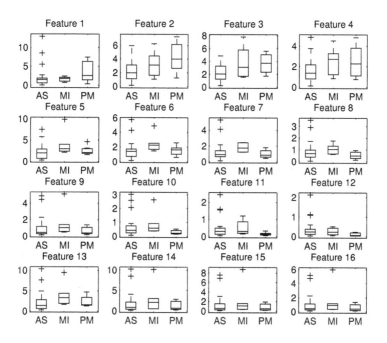

Fig. 5.27: Box and whisker plots showing results from the bispectral analysis. The 16 features are illustrated in figure 5.26. The boxes have lines at the lower quartile, median and upper quartile values. The whiskers show the extent of the data. Outliers (+) are data with values beyond the end of the whiskers.

- The waveform exhibits clear quasiperiodicity (heart beats and breathing specifically).
- The power spectral density is broad-band.

An example showing the acoustic waveform from a patient with AS is plotted along with its variance fractal dimension (VFD) trace in figure 5.28. It can be seen that the fractal dimension of the murmur is rather constant despite the large amplitude variations (crescendo-decrescendo) in the time domain. The trace was calculated by dividing the PCG signal into overlapping segments of 40 ms duration (20 ms overlap), and the VFD was calculated in each segment. Seven values along the trajectory were selected as features, see figure 5.28. The quotient between the minimum of S1 and S2 and the minimum of the five systolic values was also used as a feature to reflect the difference or strength of the murmur in relation to the heart sounds.

Estimation of fractal dimension characteristics should be based on large enough data sets [65]. This implies a trade-off between time resolution and accuracy in the estimation of the time dependent fractal dimension (similar to the uncertainty

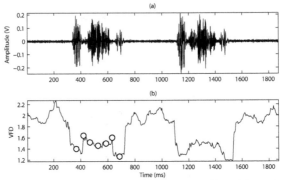

Fig. 5.28: Example of a PCG signal recorded from a patient with aortic stenosis (a) along with the variance fractal dimension trace plotted over time (b). The seven circles indicate the trace values that were used as features.

principle when calculating time-frequency representations). An example is given in figure 5.29. As the investigated signal segment does not possess self-similarity over an infinite range of scales, the self-similar properties of the segment are lost if the sliding window is too short. Similarly, if the window size is too long, the different characteristics of consecutive signal segments will be blurred together. Another reason for not using too short windows is that the number of signal amplitude increments used in the VFD algorithm must be greater than 30 to be statistically valid [124].

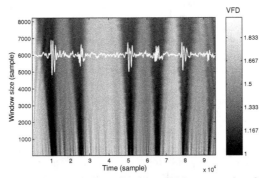

Fig. 5.29: The variance fractal dimension, encoded in gray-scale, plotted as a function of time and window size. If the window size is chosen too wide the trajectory characteristics will be blurred together while too short windows introduce errors that appear as peaks of low dimension.

Descriptive statistics for the VFD features are shown in figure 5.30. The variance is rather large, especially in the AS case, but different murmurs are quite well separated in their means. Hypothesis testing for the difference in median between the groups (the Mann-Whitney U-test) shows significant differences ($p < 0.05$) between

AS↔MI, AS↔PM and MI↔PM, respectively. Boxplots of the same data are shown in figure 5.31. In this plot, the VFD was calculated using a concatenation of all S1 segments, all S2 segments and all murmur segments from each patient. Focusing on the murmur, the trends from figure 5.30 are recognized; MI has lowest dimension, PM has highest dimension and AS is somewhere in between. The interpatient variability is mostly due to various degrees of disease severity, especially in the AS case.

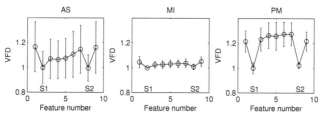

Fig. 5.30: Mean values of the variance fractal dimension at nine time instants in systole, with whiskers showing the standard deviation. The data were normalized so S1 had unit fractal dimension (for visual appearance).

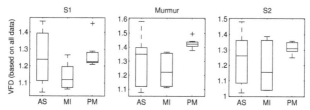

Fig. 5.31: Boxplots of the VFD when calculated for S1, murmur and S2 when concatenating all S1 data, all S2 data and all murmur data within each patient, respectively. The boxes have lines at the lower quartile, median and upper quartile values. The whiskers show the extent of the data and outliers are indicated by crosses (+).

Reconstructed state spaces

Proper embedding parameters were calculated via mutual information and Cao's method. The embedding dimension was found to be $d = 4$, which can be seen by the clearly defined knee in figure 5.32. Determination of the delay parameter was however less obvious. The mean value of the first minimum in the mutual information function was $\tau = 233 \pm 72$ samples. Since roughly half of the patients had a minimum in the vicinity of $\tau = 150$, while the other half lacked an obvious minimum in the range $\tau = 1, \ldots, 500$ samples, τ was set to 150.

Quantifying a trajectory in a four-dimensional state space is not easy. There are a few common dynamical invariants that can be used. For example, when assessing the severity of AS (section 5.1), the correlation dimension was used. Here another approach will be investigated, namely direct modeling of the trajectory's statistical distribution in state space. Povinelli et al. [191] suggest that a Gaussian mixture model (GMM) fitted to the trajectory using the Expectation-Maximization (EM) algorithm provides an efficient estimate. Here a GMM with five mixtures, see figure 5.33, was fitted to the reconstructed state space. The centers of the mixtures and the eigenvalues of their covariance matrices were used as to compactly represent the trajectory in the reconstructed state space. Even so, the five mixtures still required 40 parameters to be described. Using only five mixtures to estimate the density function of the trajectory is most likely far from enough, but the number of parameters increases rapidly with the number of mixtures. Due to the difficulty of giving an overall summary of three groups (AS, MI and PM) and 40 parameters, these results are not presented in this section. Two different sets of features were calculated based on the systolic part of the heart cycle where the heart sounds were either included in the analysis or not.

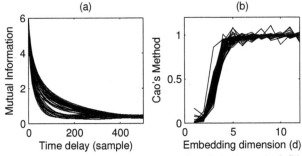

Fig. 5.32: **Auto mutual information function (a) and Cao's method (b) is used to determine the time delay and the embedding dimension d. Figure from Ahlstrom et al. [11].**

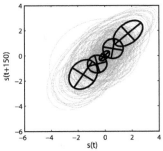

Fig. 5.33: **A reconstructed state space ($d = 2, \tau = 150$) of the systolic period from a patient with aortic stenosis. The ellipses symbolize a Gaussian mixture model with five mixtures. Note that $d = 2$ is not enough to unfold the trajectory properly. Figure from Ahlstrom et al. [11].**

Recurrence time statistics

In previous sections, high dimensional state spaces have mostly been visualized by projection into lower subspaces. The recurrence plot has been introduced to avoid this procedure by visualizing high dimensional trajectories through a two-dimensional representation of its recurrences [154]. Examples of two recurrence plots are presented in figure 5.34. Figure 5.35 shows boxplots for the RQA features obtained from data set IV. Similar to the results in section 5.1, it is clear that several of these parameters are good at separating physiological murmurs from pathological murmurs (determinism, longest diagonal line, longest vertical line and trapping time). Unfortunately, the difference between murmurs caused by AS and MI are heavily overlapping.

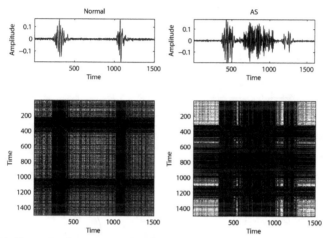

Fig. 5.34: Example of recurrence plots for a normal PCG signal and for an AS case.

5.3.2 Feature selection

Due to the large amount of features, it is not possible to perform an exhaustive search for the optimal feature set. Indeed, there are $\binom{m}{l}$ different possibilities to select l out of m features. Testing all combinations quickly becomes unfeasible. For example, finding the best subset of 14 features from the total set of 207 features requires about $1.9 \cdot 10^{21}$ tests. Instead a suboptimal feature selection algorithm can be used. Here Pudil's sequential floating forward selection (SFFS) method, which was described in section 3.10, was employed. Inclusion or rejection of features was based on the error estimate of a 1-nearest neighbor leave-one-out classifier where the performance criterion equaled the estimation error. The number of features in the final set was chosen to maximize this performance criterion while keeping the number of features as low as possible. In the end, the 207 features were reduced to 14, see figure 5.36. This feature set will be denoted the SFFS subset and it consists of the following parameters:

- *Wavelet detail*: One feature representing the end of systole.
- *Wavelet entropy*: One feature describing the information content in the high frequency range.

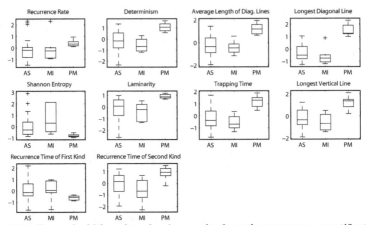

Fig. 5.35: Box and whisker plots showing results from the recurrence quantification analysis. The boxes have lines at the lower quartile, median and upper quartile values. The whiskers show the extent of the data. Outliers (+) are data with values beyond the end of the whiskers.

- *Shannon energy*: Three features in mid systole able to describe the shape and intensity of the murmur and one feature after S2 revealing the noise level.

- *S-transform*: Two features giving a collected view of the low frequency content over the heart cycle.

- *Bispectrum*: One feature indicating phase coupling and frequency content for low frequencies.

- *Reconstructed state space*: Three features describing the width of the Gaussian mixture model (probably located in the part of state space where the murmur lives), two of these belong to the largest mixture.

- *Variance fractal dimension*: Two features, one giving the amplitude normalized complexity of the murmur and the other describing S1.

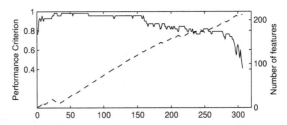

Fig. 5.36: The evolution of Pudil's sequential floating forward selection algorithm. The solid line indicates classification performance while the dashed line indicates the number of features in the present feature subset. The feature set with as few features as possible is chosen under the condition that the performance criterion is maximized. Figure from Ahlstrom et al. [11].

162

Bearing in mind that the investigated murmurs are physiological or caused by either AS or MI, the selected features are actually very reasonable. The wavelet detail represents the end of systole, where it can be used to separate holosystolic MI murmurs from physiological murmurs and AS murmurs which are of crescendo-decrescendo shape. Three Shannon energy measures represent the signal's intensity in mid systole, thereby describing the shape of the murmur in the time domain. A fractal dimension measure represents the complexity of the murmur in relation to the heart sounds. This measure can be seen as the amplitude normalized complexity of the murmur. Another fractal dimension measure, located at S1, represents the change of S1 that is usually associated with MI. Remaining features are a bit hard to explain in a physiologically meaningful way.

5.3.3 Classification

A fully connected feed-forward neural network with logarithmic sigmoid transfer functions and biased values throughout was set up to test the SFFS feature set. The number of input units was set to the nearest larger integer of the square root of the number of features in the set, the number of units in the hidden layer was set to three and the number of output units was set to two. The target values were 00 (MI), 01 (AS) or 10 (physiological murmur). Each output from the network was thresholded at 0.5 and compared to the results from a clinical echocardiography investigation. A leave-one-out approach was used for cross validation due to the limited amount of patients. For comparison, each feature extraction modality was also tested separately, i.e. the eleven feature subsets constituted by the Shannon energy, the wavelet detail, the wavelet entropy, the discretized S-transform, the eigenvalues of the time-frequency matrix, the eigentime and eigenfrequency features, the bispectral features, the two sets of GMMs, the VFD values and the RQA results. Confusion matrices showing classification results are presented in table 5.8.

Looking at the results in table 5.8, there is a tendency in several methods to classify MI and PM as AS. The total number of MI + PM patients is thirteen, and out of these patients, nine are classified incorrectly as AS using the VFD features, both Gaussian mixture models and the eigentime/eigenfrequencies, eight are classified incorrectly as AS using Shannon energy, WT entropy and bispectral features while seven are classified incorrectly as AS using the discretized S-transform, the wavelet detail and the eigenvalue features. Many of the features within each feature set are similar despite being derived from different diseases, while only a few of the features within the feature set contain the information needed to distinguish the different diseases. It is thus easy to confuse the classifier with features containing insignificant information. In the SFFS subset, only the most descriptive features from each set are used, and it is not surprising that the error rates decrease. When only considering physiological versus pathological murmurs, the percentages of correct classification according to figure 5.37 were achieved. The SFFS subset gave the best classification results while the VFD technique provided the best single-domain subset.

In this section, a straightforward multilayer perceptron network was chosen. This is a powerful nonlinear classifier, yet there are many alternatives available. In the

Table 5.8: Confusion matrices showing the classification results from the different feature subsets.

	Shannon energy			WT entropy			WT detail			ST 4x4		
	AS	MI	PM	AS	MI	PM	AS	MI	PM	AS	MI	PM
AS	17	3	3	14	7	2	15	6	2	14	8	1
MI	4	2	0	3	2	1	5	0	1	4	1	1
PM	4	1	2	5	1	1	2	4	1	3	0	4

	ST eigenvalue			ST eigenvectors			Bispectrum			GMM cycle		
	AS	MI	PM	AS	MI	PM	AS	MI	PM	AS	MI	PM
AS	15	2	6	18	4	1	14	8	1	13	3	7
MI	4	0	2	6	0	0	4	1	1	5	1	0
PM	3	1	3	3	2	2	4	1	2	4	1	2

	GMM murmur			VFD			RQA			SFFS		
	AS	MI	PM	AS	MI	PM	AS	MI	PM	AS	MI	PM
AS	15	7	1	20	2	1	8	8	7	19	2	2
MI	3	2	1	4	2	0	3	1	2	1	5	0
PM	6	0	1	5	0	2	0	3	4	0	0	7

murmur classification literature, support vector machines [114], decision trees [178], linear discriminant analysis [235] and self organizing maps [136] have been utilized. Most authors do however choose some implementation of an artificial neural network such as the multilayer perceptron network [39,46,47,113] or a grow and learn network [86, 142]. The choice of the actual classifier has not been thoroughly investigated in this chapter. However, a good classifier should be used and considerable effort needs to be spent on its design.

Ideally, data set IV should have been partitioned into four subsets. One subset for selecting and tuning the feature extraction methods, one subset for feature selection, one subset for training the classifier and a final subset for the validation. Unfortunately, this set-up requires an extensive database of PCG signals which was not available. Here, the full data set was used to design the feature extraction methods, a leave-one-out approach was used for feature selection and the same leave-one-out setup was used to train and test the classifier. This will, inevitably, affect the results in one way or another.

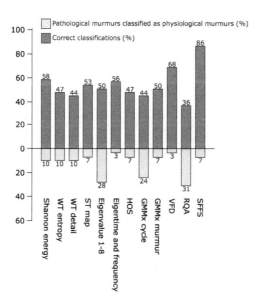

Fig. 5.37: Bar graph showing the number of correct classifications for each feature subset when used as input variables to the neural network. Also presented are the number of cases where pathological murmurs are erroneously classified as physiological. The number attached to each bar represents the exact height of the bar in percent.

6

Heart Sound Cancellation from Lung Sound Recordings

"Prediction is very difficult, especially about the future."
Niels Bohr (1885–1962)

Auscultation of lung sounds is often the first resource for detection and discrimination of respiratory diseases such as chronic obstructive pulmonary disease (COPD), pneumonia and bronchiectasis [145]. Changes in lung sounds due to disease are characterized by abnormal intensity variations or by adventitious sounds. The adventitious sounds are commonly divided into continuous sounds (wheezes) and discontinuous sounds (crackles) [215]. Wheezes are probably caused by the interaction between fluttering airway walls and the gas moving through the airways, while crackles arise due to pressure equalization when collapsed airways suddenly are opened. Diagnosis based on lung sounds is difficult, and it is desirable to remove as much obscuring noise as possible. Lung sound recordings contain noise from several sources such as heart sounds, ambient noise, muscle contractions and friction rubs. The latter can be reduced with adequate and firm microphone placement and with sound proof rooms, but heart sound noise is impossible to avoid.

There are many different methods available for heart sound cancellation from lung sound recordings. High pass filtering is often employed to reduce the influence of heart sounds. However, heart sounds and lung sounds have overlapping frequency spectra why this approach results in a loss of important signal information [41]. Other techniques employed for heart sound cancellation include wavelet based methods [41], adaptive filtering techniques [40] and fourth-order statistics [90], all resulting in reduced but still audible heart sounds [163]. Recent studies indicate that by cutting out heart sound segments and interpolating the missing data, promising results can be achieved (figure 6.1 illustrates the technique) [68, 189]. A recent method developed by Ahlstrom et al. [14] will be described in this chapter. The method is based on the idea of removing and interpolating, but the suggested signal processing techniques are fundamentally different and allow nonlinear behavior in the lung sound signal. This is an important difference since it has been indicated that lung sounds are indeed nonlinear [12, 44, 78, 233]. The evaluation in this chapter is based on data set V.

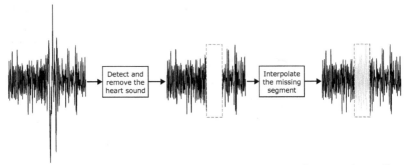

Fig. 6.1: Principle of removing a heart sound occurrence from a lung sound recording followed by interpolation of the arising gap.

6.1   Heart sound localization

Different methods for heart sound localization were described in chapter 4. Here, the method based on recurrence time statistics (section 4.3.6) will be evaluated more thoroughly in the setting of lung sound interference. Heart sounds have a transient waveform that is superpositioned/convolved upon/with lung sounds and other disturbances. Since the heart sounds and the noise originate from different sources, they have different attractors, see figure 4.27. These differences in signal dynamics are reflected in the recurrence times of the first kind ($T1$). Two interesting parameters are involved when $T1$ is used for change detection in an embedded signal; the size of the neighborhood as determined by ε (see section 3.6.2) and the width of a sliding window used to obtain time resolution.

- The window size has to be large to capture the underlying dynamics of the signal, yet it has to be small to detect fast changes. A rule of thumb is that at least a few oscillations should be included in the window.

- If ε is chosen too low, the hypersphere will be low on data and if ε is chosen too high, the hypersphere will contain misleading information from disjoint regions of the reconstructed state space. In fact, ε acts as a filter. If ε is chosen reasonably large, noise can be completely filtered out, see figure 6.2.

T1, calculated as a function of the neighborhood size ε and time, is illustrated in figure 6.3. The length of the sliding window was set to 200 ms and the overlap was excessively set to 198 ms to obtain accurate time resolution. From the figure, it is apparent that ε is a very important parameter in the detection algorithm. Interestingly, it was found that ε-values suitable for heart sound localization varied with respiration, and an adaptive algorithm for selecting a time-varying ε-value was developed. In Ahlstrom et al. [14], the slow varying envelope of the lung sound signal, determined by the low-pass filtered output of a Hilbert filter, was used. The resulting envelope had to be scaled and translated, and the choice of these parameters turned out to be quite sensitive. Figure 6.3c shows the amount of false positives and false negatives for the whole data set as a function of the translation parameter when

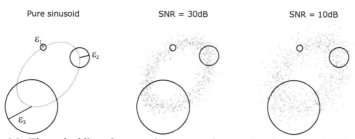

Fig. 6.2: The embedding of a pure sine wave and two noisy sine waves (SNR=30dB and SNR=10dB, respectively) are plotted in gray. The black circles represent neighborhood sizes with radii ε_1, ε_2 and ε_3. All three neighborhoods are able to estimate the period of the sinusoid in the noise free case, while a larger radius is necessary in the cases where noise is present.

fixating the scaling parameter to 0.2. Fortunately, differences between various test subjects were small, and the same parameters (*translation* = 0.11 and *scaling* = 0.2) were used throughout the whole data set. The resulting $T1(\varepsilon)$ was normalized to unity and a final threshold at 0.6 was used to detect the heart sounds (figure 6.3b). As already mentioned in section 4.3.6, an easier way to determine the time varying ε-values would be as a multiple of the standard deviation in each sliding window.

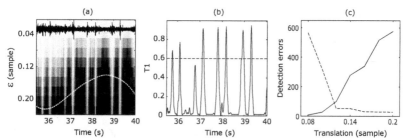

Fig. 6.3: An example showing how the recurrence time statistic indicates the location of heart sounds. Note the deep breath in the beginning of the signal. In (a), T1 is plotted over time for various ε-values, where the grey scale indicates the strength of T1. Superimposed in the figure is the PCG signal (black waveform) and the adaptive selection of ε (white). T1-values selected along the threshold are plotted in (b). The right-hand plot shows the total amount of false positives (dashed line) and false negatives (solid line) for different choices of the translation parameter used when defining the threshold.

Since the application at hand is to find and remove both S1 and S2, no attempts were made to actually classify the two sounds. Table 6.1 summarizes the results from the heart sound detection algorithm. A correct detection had to cover a whole heart sound (determined by visual inspection aided by an ECG recording). The error rates for the whole material were 4% false positives and 8% false negatives.

Table 6.1: Results from the heart sound (HS) localization step.

Subject	Number of HS	False positives	False negatives
1	208	3	9
2	174	8	23
3	168	5	17
4	220	3	34
5	140	15	11
6	298	17	5
Total	1208	51 (4%)	99 (8%)

Detection performance in the presence of adventitious lung sounds such as wheezes and crackles has not been evaluated. The attractor of wheezing sounds has a similar morphology as the attractor of heart sounds [9], and it is not inconceivable that wheezes will disturb the detection algorithm. In data set V, the measurements contained several friction rubs and one test subject had a distinct third heart sound. Most of these extra sounds were detected and removed along with S1 and S2. It is likely that explosive lung sounds like crackles will be marked by the method as well. By including extra criteria, such as interval statistics or the degree of impulsiveness, it is possible that these false detections could be avoided.

6.2 Prediction

Based on the heart sound localizations, all heart sound occurrences were simply cut out. The resulting gaps were filled with predicted lung sounds using the local nonlinear prediction scheme described in section 3.8. Six lung sound segments surrounding a removed heart sound segment was used to reconstruct the state space, and five nearest neighbors were used in the prediction. Both forward and backward prediction was used to shorten the prediction horizon by dividing the missing segment in two parts of half the size. To avoid discontinuities in the mid point, the number of predicted points was allowed to exceed past half of the segment. The two predictions were then merged in the time domain close to the midpoint at an intersection where the slopes were similar. An example of a lung sound recording after removal of the heart sounds is illustrated in figure 6.4.

The results of the predictions were hard to evaluate since the true lung sound signal was unknown in the segments that were predicted. However, the waveform similarity between predicted segments and actual lung sound data was found to be very high, showing a cross-correlation index of $CCI = 0.997 \pm 0.004$ (figure 6.5). It is, however, not surprising that the CCI-results are good since the prediction scheme exploits that trajectories in state space share the same waveform characteristics in the time domain (i.e. the prediction tries to reproduce past parts of the signal).

When trying to fill the missing gaps in the lung sound signal, the most important characteristic of the predicted data is that it appears similar to actual lung sound data. Quantitative predictions are mathematically tractable, but for nonlin-

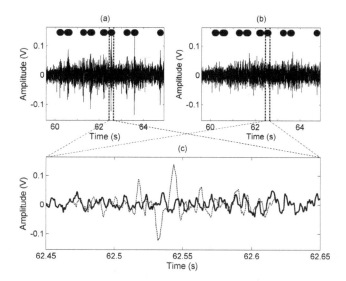

Fig. 6.4: Example of a recorded lung sound signal with heart sounds present (a) and the same signal after removing the heart sounds (b). The bars indicate heart sound detections. A zoomed in version showing the predicted lung sound (solid) and lung sound including heart sounds (dashed), is shown in (c).

ear chaotic systems, it is impossible to gain accurate results since the prediction error grows exponentially with the prediction length [118]. This is sometimes referred to as predictive hopelessness [121]. However, chaos based prediction provides qualitative results, where the general properties of the system are maintained in terms of periodicity and stability of orbits, symmetries and asymptotic behaviors, and the structure of the underlying manifold [121]. In a lung sound setting, these qualitative properties are actually very suitable.

The results were also evaluated by comparing power spectral densities between the predicted signal and the original signal where the heart sounds had been cut out (figure 6.5). Table 6.2 quantifies the differences between the original data (without heart sounds) and the predicted lung sound data, divided into four sub bands; 20 to 40 Hz, 40 to 70 Hz, 70 to 150 Hz and 150 to 300 Hz (since heart sounds have most of their energy below 300 Hz). Since the main objective of the developed method was to give high-quality auditory results, a simple complementary listening test was also performed. A skilled primary health care physician listened to the results, and the impression was that most heart sounds had been successfully replaced, but that some predictions had a slightly higher pitch than pure lung sounds.

There are a large number of methods available for heart sound cancellation from lung sound recordings. This is quite interesting since heart sound cancellation has limited clinical use (physicians are more or less able to ignore heart sounds while tuning in on lung sounds during auscultation). However, the problem at hand is

171

Table 6.2: Differences in dB/Hz (Mean ± std) between lung sounds (with removed heart sounds) and predicted lung sounds. The three periods represent the measurement phases in data set V (tidal breathing, forced respiration and breath hold).

Phase	20–40 Hz	40–70 Hz	70–150 Hz	150–300 Hz
Period 1	0.62±0.37	0.61±0.33	0.44±0.31	1.14±0.84
Period 2	2.55±0.52	3.00±0.67	2.59±0.44	2.36±0.67
Period 3	1.58±0.82	5.18±1.52	2.89±1.51	2.27±1.22
All	0.34±0.25	0.50±0.33	0.46±0.35	0.94±0.64

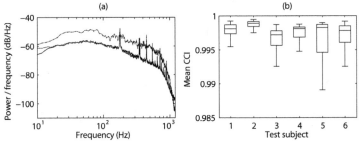

Fig. 6.5: The PSD (a) of the original signal (dash-dotted line), the original signal with heart sounds removed (solid line) and the signal where heart sounds have been replaced by nonlinear prediction (dashed line). The spectra showed are averages over all subjects and all periods. The peak at 180 Hz and its accompanying harmonics are due to a computer fan in the measurement equipment. Values of lower quartile, mean and upper quartile (boxes) of the estimated cross-correlation index (CCI) of each test subject are shown in (b).

a very intriguing engineering problem, and this is possibly one reason why it has attracted so much attention. A justification of all these methods is that automatic classifiers are confused by the heart sounds. When trying to separate different lung diseases based on lung sounds, results tend to improve after removal of the heart sounds.

The performance of the prediction algorithm in presence of adventitious lung sounds has not been evaluated. It is noteworthy that not a single heart sound cancellation method, neither the one presented here nor the ones presented in the scientific literature, has been evaluated in the presence of spontaneous artifacts. Most methods have actually been investigated in a controlled (silent) environment and on healthy subjects in known cardiac (no additive sounds or murmurs) and respiratory (no crackles or wheezes) states [77]. This presents some very likely problems when these methods are used in the clinic. If heart sounds are dampened, will crackles be dampened as well? If heart sounds are removed and the missing gaps are filled using interpolation, will there be enough surrounding data to facilitate the prediction when long duration murmur segments have been removed? What happens with the heart sound localization algorithms when the heart sounds are obscured by wheezes? Many questions remain to be answered before any of these techniques can be introduced in a clinical setting.

7

Cardiovascular Time Intervals

"Whenever I feel blue, I start breathing again."
Lyman Frank Baum (1856–1919)

Altered cardiovascular time intervals are indicative of diseases such as heart failure and valvular lesions [236]. These changes are however measured as trends over long time scales. There are also faster variations which reflect physiological processes such as blood pressure and breathing. These short-time effects will be investigated in this chapter, especially with a noninvasive, non-occlusive and non-intrusive monitoring device in mind. Time intervals relevant for this chapter are summarized in this introduction and illustrated in figure 7.1. Included are the pre-ejection period (PEP), the left ventricular ejection time (LVET), the isovolumic contraction time (IVCT), the electromechanical activation time (EMAT), the vessel transit time (VTT) and the pulse wave transit time (PTT). PEP, IVCT and LVET are not explicitly used in this chapter why their descriptions are rather brief. For completeness, they are however included in the figure and mentioned in the text.

Electromechanical activation time (EMAT)
EMAT is measured from the Q-wave in the ECG to the initial rise in left ventricular pressure, and reflects the electromechanical activity required for the left ventricle to close the mitral valve. S1 can be used to mark the end point of EMAT if the pressure curve is unavailable. Factors affecting EMAT include conduction defects, the integrity of the mitral valve and the rate of rise of ventricular pressure [236].

Isovolumic contraction time (IVCT)
This measure is derived as the time difference between S1 and the upstroke in an aortic pressure curve. Since it is cumbersome to measure aortic pressure, a carotid pulse recording is often used instead. A decrease in IVCT suggests a greater velocity of cardiac contraction [236].

Pre-ejection period (PEP) and left ventricular ejection time (LVET)
PEP comprises EMAT and IVCT, thus ranging from electrical activation of the heart to the opening of the aortic valve. Factors influencing PEP include preload, afterload, ventricular contractility, valve lesions, ischemic heart disease, hypertension, cardiomyopathy, inotropic drugs and conduction defects [236]. For practical reasons, PEP is usually measured from the Q-wave or the R-peak in the ECG to

173

S2 minus LVET. LVET is in turn measured as the time interval ranging from the upstroke of an aortic pressure curve to the incisura of the same pressure curve, see figure 7.1.

There is some controversy regarding the relationship between the constituents of PEP. Some state that EMAT remains constant under the influence of a variety of mechanisms including changes in contractility, preload, afterload and heart rate while all these factors affect ICVT (which consequently becomes highly correlated to PEP) [152]. Yet again, others have claimed that the correlation between PEP and heart rate is mostly due to changes in EMAT [239].

Changes in PEP and LVET are often related, where a decrease in PEP is accompanied by an increase in LVET and vice versa. In fact, the PEP/LVET ratio is the most widely used time interval index for assessing left ventricular dysfunction [209]. Due to interaction and coupling in the cardiovascular system, this ratio reflects changes in preload, afterload and contractility, which in turn reflect pathologic conditions such as heart failure and valvular lesions.

Vessel transit time (VTT)
The vessel transit time is the time it takes for the arterial pulse pressure wave to travel from the aortic valve to the periphery. The R-peak in the ECG is often used as an estimate of aortic valve closure, not because it is very accurate, but because it is robust to noise and easy to pinpoint in time. A more accurate onset time could however be determined as the upstroke of the aortic pressure curve. The peripheral site could, for example, be the finger where the arrival time of the pulse can be

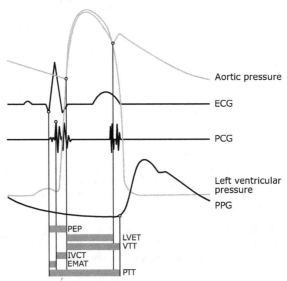

Fig. 7.1: Illustration of cardiovascular time intervals in relation to the cardiac cycle.

measured by a photoplethysmograph. The main factors influencing VTT are heart rate and vessel compliance [51].

The more rigid the wall of the artery, the faster the wave travels. VTT is therefore used as an index of arterial stiffness and an indicator of atherosclerosis [131]. VTT has also been suggested as an indirect estimate of beat-to-beat blood pressure [43,69, 150,165,186]. Since VTT is dependent on the distance that the pulse wave travels, the velocity is usually calculated instead. Arterial distances measured over the body surface are however inaccurate why velocity calculations are cumbersome.

Pulse wave transit time (PTT)
PTT is the time from electrical activation of the heart to the arrival of the arterial pressure pulse at a peripheral site [115]. The general definition of PTT is thus the sum of PEP and VTT, see figure 7.1. In practise PTT is measured as the time difference between the R-peak in the ECG and the upstroke of a photoplethysmographic curve measured on the finger. Factors reflected in PTT are the same as in PEP and VTT, respectively.

The long term variations described so far are not the focus of this chapter, instead the short term effects will be investigated in more detail. The cardiovascular system continuously adapts itself to secure the oxygen delivery to the body, see section 2.1.4. These beat-by-beat adjustments cause short term fluctuations in the cardiovascular time intervals, where both respiration and blood pressure changes are visible. An introductory example showing how EMAT varies as a function of respiration and blood pressure is illustrated in figure 7.2.

This chapter is restricted to cardiovascular time intervals as measured via ECG, PCG and photoplethysmography (PPG). The main consequence of such a setup is that the aortic pressure curve is not available. This means that the upstroke of aortic pressure has to be estimated by S1 and that the incisura has to be estimated by S2.

7.1 Continuous monitoring of blood pressure changes

The velocity of the arterial pressure pulse depends on blood pressure why numerous attempts have been made to estimate blood pressure based on the pulse wave velocity [43, 69, 150, 165, 186]. Although it may be difficult to extract an absolute value of blood pressure without regular calibrations, tracking of changes in systolic blood pressure seems feasible [13, 43].

Already in the 1920s, the velocity of the pulse wave and its effect on arterial extensibility was investigated by Bramwell and Hill [36]. As blood pressure increases, arterial compliance decreases and the pulse wave travels faster (VTT decreases). Different analytical expressions describing the relationship between VTT and vessel dynamics have been presented. Most common are Moens-Korteweg's [43], Womersley's [69] and Bramwell-Hill's [36] formulas. Provided that some variables are

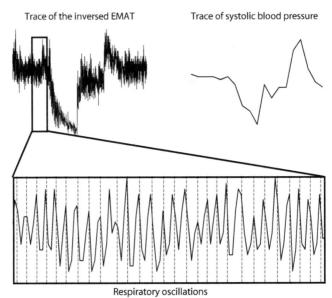

Fig. 7.2: Introductory example of the electromechanical activation time (EMAT) measured over a time period of 20 min. The inverse trace (beat-by-beat) of EMAT (top left), measured from the R-peak in an ECG to S1, closely resembles the systolic blood pressure trace (top right). Enlarging a small part of the trace reveals the respiratory oscillations. The dotted vertical lines are breaths as determined by a respiration reference. Figure from Ahlstrom et al. [15].

considered constant, all of these expressions model the inverse relationship between VTT and blood pressure by a linear regression. Moen-Korteweg's formula, see equation 7.1, was used by Chen et al. [43] to relate VTT to the dimensions of the vessel and the distensibility of the vessel wall. v is the pulse wave velocity, E is the elastic modulus of the vessel, ρ is the density of blood, a is the wall thickness and d is the interior diameter of the vessel. The elastic modulus increases exponentially with increasing blood pressure according to equation 7.2. E_0 is the elastic modulus at zero pressure, P is the blood pressure (Pa) and γ is a coefficient ranging from 0.016 to 0.018 (Pa^{-1}), depending on the particular vessel [43].

$$v = \sqrt{\frac{Ea}{d\rho}} \qquad (7.1)$$

$$E = E_0 e^{\gamma P} \qquad (7.2)$$

By combining equations 7.1 and 7.2, and setting the velocity $v = K/T$, equation 7.3 is obtained. K indicates the distance for the pulse wave to transit within time T. If the changes in a, d and E_0 are considered negligible or slow, the first term on the right-hand side of equation 7.3 can be regarded as a constant during a short time period. Taking the derivative with respect to T results in equation 7.4. From equation 7.4 it can be seen that a pressure change has an inverse linear relationship to T.

$$P = \frac{1}{\gamma} \left(ln \frac{d\rho K^2}{aE_0} - 2lnT \right) \qquad (7.3)$$

$$\frac{\partial P}{\partial T} = -\frac{2}{T\gamma} \qquad (7.4)$$

For practical reasons, the pulse wave transit time is often measured as the time between the R-peak of the ECG and the onset of the peripheral pulse detected via the photoplethysmogram of a pulse oximeter ($PTT = PEP + VTT$). High correlations between PTT and systolic blood pressure (SBP) have been reported, but the agreement with diastolic blood pressure is weak [17]. To improve the correlation between PTT and SBP further, it has been suggested that PEP should be excluded from PTT. After all, Moens-Korteweg's theoretical framework only accounts for the time that the pulse wave travels through the vessels. This suggestion have, however, been disputed since PEP seems to be an important contributor to the correlation between PTT and SBP [150, 165].

PEP has been recognized as an estimate of preload [164]. As preload is affected by blood volume (pressure) it is conceivable that PEP is modulated by blood pressure. Hypothesizing that this is the case, PEP and VTT are both varying with blood pressure and their combined effect should make blood pressure fluctuations more evident. This approach will, however, violate the direct relationship between transit times and blood pressure suggested by Moens-Korteweg's equation. The remainder of section 7.1 will be spent investigating PTT and PEP. Data set I, see page 6, was used in these investigations. Since a carotid pulse recording was not available in data set I, the EMAT parameter was used as a surrogate to PEP (preload is one of the determinants of EMAT, so this discrepancy should not affect the results greatly). To quickly recapitulate the material in data set I, it consists of five phases; resting, hypotension, resting, hypertension and resting. Lower body negative pressure (LBNP) was applied to invoke hypotension [173] and isometric muscle contraction was used to invoke hypertension [69].

The content in this section on monitoring of blood pressure changes is based on a combination of the results from Ahlstrom et al. [13] and Ahlstrom et al. [15].

7.1.1 Extraction of transit times

Three different transit times were calculated: PTT, EMAT(MR) extracted with the multi resolution S1 localizer (see section 4.2.1) and EMAT(EA) extracted with the ECG-gated ensemble averaging approach (see section 4.2.1). PEP and EMAT were thus defined as (source signal in parenthesis):

PTT = Time from R-peak (ECG) to onset of peripheral pulse (PPG)

EMAT = Time from R-peak (ECG) to S1 (PCG)

S1 was detected as outlined in section 4.2.1, and the R-peak in the ECG was detected by simple thresholding. To find the onset of the peripheral pulse, the PPG signal was segmented into heart cycles using the RR-intervals [13]. The onset was then marked as the first local minimum to the left of the maximum value in each segment. The detected onset points were used for creating continuous (beat-by-beat) traces of the three transit times, see figures 7.3 and 7.4. In cases where the algorithms failed to detect accurate onsets, the incorrect detections were removed manually for PTT, whereas incorrect detections in EMAT were removed based on the same criteria that were used on page 103.

Blood pressure recordings and transit times contained fluctuations with frequency content higher than that of realistic pressure changes. These were removed with a low-pass filter (5th order zero-phase Butterworth filter with a cut-off frequency corresponding to 0.02 Hz assuming a heart rate of one beat per second). An example of the three transit time traces along with intermittent measurements of SBP is shown in figure 7.3. An immediate observation is that EMAT(EA) provides significantly higher transit time values compared to EMAT(MR). This is due to the fact that the ensemble averaging approach marked S1 occurrences when the template was abreast of S1 while the multi resolution approach located the first peak within S1.

7.1.2 Agreement between transit times and blood pressure

PTT as well as EMAT was negatively correlated to SBP (based on transit times extracted from data set I), see table 7.1. The baseline levels were analyzed separately for the three measurement phases (the resting phases were put together and analyzed as one). Higher baseline values were found during hypotension, as compared to resting conditions, for both PTT and EMAT (table 7.2). For hypertension, although weak, an opposite tendency was seen. The results for PTT agree with several studies [17,43,69,150,165,168]. However, PEP has been reported to show great interpatient variability with positive as well as negative correlations with SBP [179,187]. This indicates that EMAT is a more stable time interval compared to PEP when assessing blood pressure changes. However, these results need to be confirmed in a study where PEP, EMAT and the isovolumic contraction time are derived on a large amount of patients with conformed reference methods, not from the ECG and PCG alone.

The transit time baseline values from hypertension showed a small (nonsignificant) decrease as compared with resting conditions. This surprisingly small decrease might derive from the isometric muscle contraction. This provocation can only be maintained for a shorter time, it affects the peripheral resistance by direct mechanical compression and its effect on SBP is not fully clear [103]. Regarding PTT, another explanation is provided by Moens-Korteweg's formula (equation 7.3) which states that SBP and PTT are exponentially related. Variations in the high pressure region will thus give a smaller change in transit time compared to variations in the low pressure region. Regarding PEP, and possibly EMAT as well, recent findings suggest that PEP is rather reflecting fluid responsiveness and that the correlation to

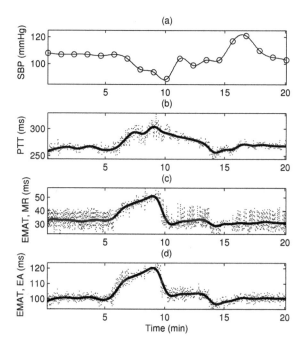

Fig. 7.3: Example of the inverse relationship between SBP (a) and PTT (b) in a test subject. The solid line shows the low frequency changes in the data. Corresponding curves for EMAT(MR) and EMAT(EA) are shown in (c) and (d), respectively. The two provocation phases are clearly seen in the top plot as hypotension between 5 and 10 minutes and as hypertension after 15 minutes. The time resolution is one sample per obtained blood pressure reading (a) and one sample per heartbeat (b, c and d). Faster variations are mainly respiratory fluctuations.

blood pressure is a secondary effect [24]. This could explain EMAT's agreement to hypovolemia (induced by LBNP) as well as the modest reaction to isometric muscle contraction.

EMAT accounted for a larger percentage of PTT during the hypotension phase. Calculated via the ensemble averaging approach, EMAT corresponded to 41% of PTT during hypotension compared to 36% during rest and hypertension. This is an additional indication that PEP is highly affected by changes in blood volume. It also demonstrates that PTT should not be used as a substitute for pulse wave velocity for assessment of arterial stiffness (if PEP is not constant, it will violate Moens-Korteweg's formula). This latter finding is in agreement with the results from Payne et al. [179].

As already mentioned, the inclusion of PEP when using PTT to estimate SBP is still actively debated. Since SBP is dependent on both vascular and ventricular

179

Table 7.1: Correlation between the three transit times and SBP (all measurement phases together, MR = multi resolution, EA = ensemble averaging).

Subject	PTT	EMAT(MR)	EMAT(EA)
1	-0.80	-0.83	-0.86
2	-0.80	-0.91	-0.85
3	-0.92	-0.44	-0.58
4	-0.79	-0.70	-0.73
5	-0.78	-0.74	-0.75
6	-0.73	-0.67	-0.74
7	-0.85	-0.76	-0.77
8	-0.76	-0.73	-0.84
Mean±std	0.80 ± 0.06	0.72 ± 0.14	0.76 ± 0.09

Table 7.2: Baseline values (ms), mean ± std, of the three transit times for each measurement phase (MR = multi resolution, EA = ensemble averaging).

Phase	PTT	EMAT(MR)	EMAT(EA)
Hypotension	282.1 ± 22.4	49.6 ± 12.5	115.1 ± 9.6
Resting	260.7 ± 18.9	30.1 ± 8.0	94.4 ± 4.4
Hypertension	254.4 ± 18.9	29.0 ± 9.3	90.8 ± 4.9

contraction, it comes as no surprise that PTT, a composite of both vascular and cardiac activity, is correlated to SBP. The current standpoint is that PEP should not be included when trying to estimate blood pressure [43,179], however, it should be included if only changes in SBP are sought [13,179]. The results presented in this section clearly showed that EMAT, which is a subset of PEP, was correlated to SBP. This fact supports the hypothesis that PEP should be included when estimating blood pressure changes from transit times.

7.2 Respiration monitoring

Monitoring of respiration is a fundamental component in fields such as intensive care, postoperative care, anesthesia and neonatal care. Nonetheless, no technical method yet exists that satisfies demands on sensitivity, specificity, patient safety and user friendliness [116]. Non-obstructing techniques able to extract respiration rate in combination with other monitoring parameters are often preferred to air-flow based sensors. An example of such a solution is transthoracic impedance plethysmography, which is integrated with the ECG electrodes.

It is well known that blood pressure decreases during inspiration. The transit times, which are modulated by a blood pressure synchronous component, might thus be modulated by a respiration synchronous component as well. In fact, it has been demonstrated that PEP is lengthened during inspiration [150,165,184], and since PEP is part of PTT, it is reasonable to believe that PTT is also lengthened during inspiration. Applications of this respiration synchronous component of the PTT have so far been restricted to grading respiratory effort in connection with obstructive sleep apnea [185, 186]. The remainder of this section will be spent investigating and discussing the effects of respiration on PTT and PEP. As in section 7.1, the EMAT parameter will be used as a substitute to PEP. The content in this section is a combination of the results reported in Ahlstrom et al. [15] and in Johansson et al. [115].

7.2.1 Agreement between transit times and respiration

Using data set I, 2326 respiratory cycles from eight test subjects were analyzed. The three transit times that were extracted in the previous section were here re-used in the respiratory setting. An example of the three transit time traces is presented in figure 7.4.

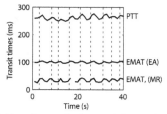

Fig. 7.4: Typical transit time traces during rest (normotension). Dashed lines are expirations as detected by the respiration reference. The top trace represents PTT, followed by EMAT(EA) and EMAT(MR) at the bottom. The missing value in the bottom trace is due to a detection error.

The mean amplitude of the respiratory variation is presented in table 7.3. The amplitude was defined as half the difference between the maximum and minimum transit time value within each reference respiratory cycle. Reference respiratory cycles were set as the regions between expiration marks in the respiration reference. In the previous section, it was noted that the transit time baselines responded inversely to the provocations invoking hypo- or hypertension, respectively (table 7.2). Despite these blood pressure induced changes, the respiration amplitudes were not significantly affected. This indicates that despite coarse physiological provocations, the respiratory synchronous fluctuations in the transit times remain intact.

Table 7.3: Mean amplitudes (ms), mean $\pm$ std, of the respiratory variation for the three transit times (MR = multi resolution, EA = ensemble averaging).

Phase	PTT	EMAT(MR)	EMAT(EA)
Hypotension	3.5 ± 3.4	1.4 ± 1.4	2.2 ± 1.5
Resting	4.2 ± 3.9	1.4 ± 1.2	1.5 ± 0.8
Hypertension	4.0 ± 3.5	1.0 ± 0.8	1.1 ± 0.7

The number of false positive and false negative breath detections for PTT and the two EMAT measures are presented in table 7.4. A breath was assumed correct if there was exactly one local minimum in the transit time trace during the reference respiratory cycle. A false positive was registered if there was more than one minimum and a false negative if there were no minima. Best results in breath detection were seen for PTT in the normotension phase with a total error rate of 12%. The error rates were significantly increased for the hypotension and hypertension phases. In general, false positive errors dominated over false negative errors. The higher error rates found during the blood pressure provocations are probably explained by unstable physiological conditions. In the EMAT cases, there was also additional acoustic noise introduced by the LBNP device. Comparing the two approaches of determining EMAT, ensemble averaging gave slightly better results. In the hypotension phase, where noise from the LBNP device heavily influenced the PCG signal, EMAT(EA) resulted in a 13% increase in the amount of correct breath detections. This is a direct consequence entailed by the more accurate S1 detector.

Table 7.4: False positive (FP) and false negative (FN) breath detections (%) in the three transit times for each measurement phase (MR = multi resolution, EA = ensemble averaging).

Phase	PTT		EMAT(MR)		EMAT(EA)	
	FP	FN	FP	FN	FP	FN
Hypotension	30	4	58	2	39	8
Resting	8	4	20	4	19	1
Hypertension	14	2	22	6	21	4

The transit time values were normalized to the region [0 1], and mean values of these patterns were calculated to obtain information about the direction of change and phase lag between respiration and the transit time traces. For all three phases (hypotension, hypertension and resting) it was clear that PTT as well as EMAT decreased as a first response (five heartbeats) to expiration, see figure 7.5. It is also worth noticing that the hypothesis of increasing transit times following inspiration seems correct, both in normotension and during blood pressure provocations.

An interesting finding in this section was that the reported respiratory synchronous fluctuations in PEP [150, 165, 184] are also present in EMAT. To measure these fluctuations, it is however necessary to use accurate localization of S1. Further, since respiration directly affects the circulation by reducing systolic blood pressure during inspiration, a reduced mean blood pressure gives rise to a longer VTT [115]. In combination with the respiratory modulation of EMAT, simple superposition explains why the most robust mean respiratory amplitudes were found in PTT.

7.3 Additional comments

Accurate continuous blood pressure monitoring can only be achieved via an intra-arterial pressure sensor. Catheter insertion is however always associated with a certain risk of embolism, infections or injuries of peripheral nerves. Despite these risks, invasive blood pressure monitoring is the only continuous technique which is accepted for clinical use today. Non-invasive estimates of the pressure curve are usually based on the vascular unloading technique. However, these techniques suf-

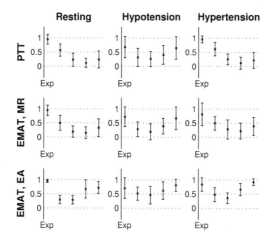

Fig. 7.5: Mean and standard deviation values of the normalized transit time patterns for the five consecutive heartbeats after expiration (MR = multi resolution, EA = ensemble averaging).

fer from insufficient accuracy and stability. Since an externally applied pressure is required, they are also occlusive, which in the long run can cause tissue trauma. The occlusion itself also means stress for the patient, a condition which undoubtedly affects the blood pressure. When it comes to non-invasive and non-occlusive continuous blood pressure monitoring, available methods are restricted to transit time modeling. This technique is not yet accurate enough to monitor the absolute value of blood pressure, but tracking of blood pressure changes is achievable.

Similar difficulties apply to respiration monitoring. Direct methods are accurate but also very intrusive since the sensor is attached to the airways in one way or another. There are, unfortunately, no good alternative indirect methods (not based on air flow) available. It would have been interesting to compare transit time based methods with other indirect measures such as transthoracic impedance (TTI) or respiratory sinus arrhythmia (RSA) derived from ECG. Such a comparison is however left for future studies. It should be noted that both TTI and RSA can be measured with the same sensors as was used in this chapter. Combining information from many sources is thus conceivable to improve both accuracy and robustness.

A noninvasive and non-intrusive multi-sensor device, fitted into a simple chest belt, would be able to monitor ECG and PCG as well as be able to estimate respiration and blood pressure fluctuations. Such a device would be very useful in home health care as well as in exercise testing, sport sciences and certain clinical applications. A typical clinical application is the investigation of sleeping disorders, where noninvasive, non-obstructive and non-intrusive sensors are necessary in order not to disturb the patient's sleeping patterns [185].

8

Complementary Remarks and Future Aspects

"Doubt is not a pleasant condition, but certainty is absurd."
Voltaire (1694–1778)

In a small pilot study performed by our research group[1] in 2002, interviews with primary health care physicians revealed that the most interesting task for an intelligent stethoscope was classification of heart murmurs, especially to distinguish physiological murmurs from pathological murmurs. These interviews formed the basis of our bioacoustic research and greatly influenced the questions addressed in this book. This chapter is a collection of ideas, thoughts and preliminary results regarding our current research and its continuation.

8.1 Areas of application

Evaluation of patients with heart disease is a complex task, where auscultation provides one piece of the puzzle. Therefore, a PCG based decision support system should not be seen as a tool capable of replacing clinicians or other diagnostic techniques, but rather as a mean to quantify and clarify information from the PCG signal. By alerting the auscultator when abnormal sounds are present in the signal, or by helping to decide whether a murmur is innocent or not, much could be gained in form of more accurate early diagnoses. This is, in my opinion, the main area of application for an intelligent stethoscope. In the primary care, when deciding which patients that need special care, an intelligent stethoscope could really make a difference. Another application of interest is to follow the progress of a disease. If the disease state is monitored by PCG signal analysis, recurrent echocardiographic examinations in the clinic could be less frequent. This topic is directly related to the aim of making auscultation more objective.

Just as in the human health care system, there is a primary health care and a specialized/centralized care in veterinary medicine as well. This implies that the main areas of application for an intelligent stethoscope are the same regardless if the patient is human or an animal. AS and MI are the most important structural

---

[1]Physiological Measurements, Department of Biomedical Engineering, Linköping University, Sweden (http://www.imt.liu.se).

heart diseases in dogs and especially classification of physiological murmurs from pathological murmurs is of great interest. There is, however, an important difference between humans and animals concerning the interesting stage of the disease. In humans, surgical correction is generally performed well before the disease causes any secondary changes. In this case it is important to find the disease at an early stage. In animals on the other hand, cardiac surgery is very rare and the important stage of the disease is when it is time to start a medical treatment. This usually occurs at a more severe disease stage. This means that algorithms developed for humans needs to be adjusted to be used in veterinary science and vice versa.

Cardiac imaging by means of echocardiography or magnetic resonance imaging (MRI) are diagnostic techniques which outperform auscultation and phonocardiography when it comes to accurate assessment of cardiac function. These techniques do however require expensive, often immobile, equipment and requires specially trained clinicians. Auscultation with an intelligent stethoscope is usable by a broader spectrum of clinicians and investigations can be performed both in the clinic or at home. A competitive technique is the portable ultrasound equipment [201]. In due time, such mobile echocardiography devices will inevitably be equipped with computer vision software able to guide even an inexperienced sonographer so that high quality images are obtained.

8.2 Limitations

8.2.1 Clinical validation

Many of the methods presented in this book have not been clinically validated. All methods have been developed and tested on data acquired from either test subjects, patients or dogs, but clinical validation on a large number of unseen human patients is necessary before any final conclusions can be drawn from the results. In chapter 4, the developed S1 localization algorithm was designed based on simulated data and verified on healthy test subjects. The regression models were however not tested on patients. In chapter 5, many algorithms were designed and adjusted based on data from dogs and a leave-one-out approach was used to verify the classification results, but the methods need to be validated on human patients. In section 5.3, the same data set was used for feature selection as well as for leave-one-out classification why a new unseen material of patients is needed to verify the results. Finally, in chapter 6, the heart sound cancellation method was developed and tested on healthy test subjects while the main area of application would be patients with lung disease.

8.2.2 Computational complexity

Many of the methods used in this book suffer from high computational burden. This is a problem since the software is supposed to be implemented in a portable intelligent stethoscope, preferably in real time. It is however difficult to assess the actual performance limitations of the used signal processing methods since they were never designed to be quick or efficient. A number of potential speed-ups are:

- MATLAB was used to implement all algorithms, but using a lower level language would improve the performance.

- Fast nearest neighbor routines are available, but currently a very simple search routine is used.

- A sliding window approach is often used to gain time resolution. The reconstructed state space is nearly identical between iterations due to the overlap between segments, and this fact is not exploited.

A fundamentally different bottle-neck is the fact that some calculations are non-causal. For instance, many of the features in chapter 5 were derived as averages over all available heart cycles. In most cases this could be dealt with by only using old data. Accumulated statistics could then be used to increase the accuracy of the output as more data become available. In either way, real-time performance is not that important in a classification situation. As long as the result is presented within consultation time it will be fast enough.

8.2.3 Stationarity

Stationarity is an underlying assumption in many of the methods used in this book. Interestingly, a time series can be considered both stationary and nonstationary depending on the time scale of interest. For example, the heart rate of a resting person is often treated as homogeneous over several minutes. Longer recordings such as a 24-hour Holter ECG does however cover slower variations such as the circadian rhythm and can no longer be considered stationary. The PCG signal is definitely nonstationary when a single heart cycle is under investigation. If the data is acquired over a longer period of time, the heart cycle repeats itself in a nearly periodic manner why such recordings can be considered stationary. In the data sets used in this book, the PCG signals typically consist of about ten heart cycles. Such a time window is short enough so that really slow variations can be ignored. It is however not long enough to account for faster variations due to respiration. This latter issue is dealt with by asking the patients to hold their breath. In conclusion, stationarity is an awkward quality to guarantee and in this work, rather simple countermeasures have been used to relieve nonstationarity issues. This matter should definitely be investigated more carefully in the future.

8.2.4 Chaos or noise?

Turbulence itself has been shown to be chaotic [200], and due to the strong interaction between fluid flow and its induced sound field [241], it is reasonable to believe that the chaotic behavior is preserved in the PCG signal. The greatest problems when trying to determine if a time series is chaotic are that the results are almost always open for interpretation, that nearly noise free data is required and that the amount of data should be large. In the early days of nonlinear signal analysis, convergence of the correlation dimension was interpreted as evidence of low dimensional deterministic chaos. The convincing scaling region in figure 5.7 would have been proof enough. After the finding that filtered noise can also demonstrate converging correlation dimensions, the necessity of surrogate data tests was stressed. Again, surrogate tests of the PCG signal indicate that the data should be nonlinear. The strength of such a test is however limited to the manufacturing of the surrogate data. In the end, it might not be that important whether the PCG signal consists of colored noise or chaos. Of more interest is the possibility to quantify heart diseases using chaos based signal processing.

8.3 Future work

8.3.1 Creating a murmur map

In the literature, heart murmurs are usually described by means of pressures and flows within the heart. The task for the auscultating physician is to solve the inverse problem and translate the sounds into pressure and flow fluctuations and further into physiological events. As outlined in chapter 3, findings in dynamical systems theory allow this inverse problem to be partially solved. Using Takens' delay embedding theorem, the recorded sound signal can be used to reconstruct or estimate the flow conditions from where the sound once sprung. In this book, certain invariant measures such as the fractal dimension have been used to describe the reconstructed dynamics. However, a lot of information is thrown away when summarizing all available information into one single measure. Hypothesizing that the embedded signal really resides on a manifold in the reconstructed state space, it would be very interesting to investigate how the geometry of this manifold changes as different diseases influence the cardiovascular dynamics.

To test the eligibility of these ideas, a naive algorithm was implemented and evaluated on the 29 patients with innocent murmurs or murmurs caused by AS in data set IV. The recorded PCG signals were embedded in a reconstructed state space using Takens' delay embedding theorem with $d = 5$ and $\tau = 5.5$ ms. Each embedding was looked upon as a point set, and the Bhattacharyya distance [225] between their respective distributions was calculated. This provided a distance matrix containing information about how far away each embedding was from every other embedding. Based on the distance matrix, it is possible to construct a map showing the relationship between different patients. Here multidimensional scaling was used to create the map, but many alternatives are available. As can be seen in figure 8.1, patients with similar AS severity tends to cluster (the classification was based on the AHA guidelines [30]). Actually, if the first dimension of the multidimensional scaling results is plotted against AS severity, a correlation coefficient of $R = 0.80$ is achieved, see figure 8.1. It is important to realize that it is a very naive approach to use the Bhattacharyya distance on these kinds of data. However, the example does indicate the potential of the concept. In fact, the R-value is better than the ones obtained in section 5.1.

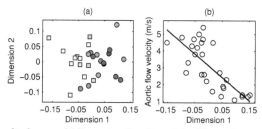

Fig. 8.1: Results from multidimensional scaling of the Bhattacharyya distances where the patients with considerable AS (boxes) and the patients with mild or no AS (circles) group themselves into separate subgroups (a). The gray scale represents the aortic flow velocity where black is 0 m/s and white is about 5.5 m/s. The correspondence between dimension 1 and AS severity is illustrated in (b).

8.3.2 Feature extraction, classification and beyond

The standpoint of this book is that the most important step in any classification system is the extraction and selection of descriptive features. A different approach is to present large sets of nearly raw data, such as a full joint time-frequency matrix, to the classifier. In this approach, the recognition system also contains a feature extractor, but the feature extractor is incorporated in the internal structure of the classifier. Perhaps this alternative route to classification is even more accessible. After all, it seems like this is the way the human brain is operating [97].

Along the same line of thought, dimension reduction could be applied to large data sets such as joint time-frequency matrices or embedding matrices. Classical linear methods for dimension reduction include principal component analysis and multidimensional scaling. However, if the data can not be accurately summarized by linear combinations, these techniques are insufficient. A simple example is provided by the three dimensional helix whose one-dimensional structure cannot be discovered by linear methods. Instead of finding the most important linear subspace from a set of data points (like in principal component analysis), nonlinear parameterizations can be sought. Many of these manifold learning techniques are based on a distance matrix (like multidimensional scaling in the last section). In principle, the difference compared to multidimensional scaling is the way that distances are calculated. Instead of measuring a global distance (a straight line through space), the distance is calculated by summing up local distances as one moves from one point to another (i.e. we are only allowed to travel from point a to point b via other data points located in between). A problem associated with these techniques is whether the data really resides on a manifold and if so, whether the manifold is sampled dense enough to create a reliable distance matrix. A simple experiment was conducted to test the validity of this idea. The averaged joint time-frequency matrices were calculated with the S-transform for each patient in data set IV having either an innocent murmur or a murmur caused by AS. The size of the matrices was reduced to 100×200 data values to reduce the memory requirements, resulting in a 20000-dimensional feature space. The dimension of this data set was reduced by locally linear embedding [199], and the resulting two-dimensional space is illustrated in figure 8.2. The interesting aspect of both this approach and the one presented in the last section is that the algorithms find structure in the data without any guidance. Here 29 examples of a 20000-dimensional data representation are presented to a black box and out comes a two-dimensional map indicating the severity of the disease. Results from this experiment should however be interpreted as is. After all, no particular thought was put into the construction of the high-dimensional feature space. Comparing the first resulting dimension with the aortic flow velocity, a correlation coefficient of $R = 0.82$ was obtained. Again, a simple experiment has showed that nonlinear signal processing provides very valuable tools. It should be noted that this example does not make use of nonlinearities in the data (the S-transform is linear). It does however deal with nonstationarity in a straightforward manner. Perhaps it would be fruitful to use the Hilbert-Huang transform [106] to compute the feature matrix because this technique is able to treat both nonlinear and nonstationary data at the same time.

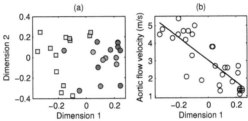

Fig. 8.2: **Results from dimensionality reduction by locally linear embedding where the patients with considerable AS (boxes) and the patients with mild or no AS (circles) group themselves into separate subgroups (a). The gray scale represents the aortic flow velocity where black is 0 m/s and white is about 5.5 m/s. The correspondence between dimension 1 and AS severity is illustrated in (b).**

8.3.3 The forest and the trees

It is all too easy to get lost in the forest if you focus on the trees, and however tempting it is to use nifty processing algorithms, it is important to remember the rest of the system. An intelligent stethoscope does not only contain software connected to a sound sensor. It also needs a high-end amplifier, an AD-converter able to send accurate data to a sufficiently fast DSP chip via a wide enough data bus, an intelligible user interface, all packed up in a compact and robust cover. As of today, the Meditron electronic stethoscope has been used to acquire the PCG signal. This stethoscope can be directly connected to a computer via a sound card. In the computer, all the necessary processing power is readily available. Within the scope of this book, this setup has been more than adequate to develop signal processing methods. However, all of these design issues have to be solved in a future auscultation system where a graphical display, built in memory, wireless data transmission, adaptive noise reduction etc. should all be fitted into a small portable device.

Speaking of sensors, an interesting extension of the work in this book would be to incorporate multi-sensor data. The magnitude of different components in the PCG signal varies with the measurement location, so by determining the puncta maxima of a murmur, a fair indication of its origin is obtained. By using multiple sensors in parallel, this difference in intensity could be used as a parameter in a classification system. Further uses could be to derive time differences between the different signals and, by using this information, calculate an estimate of the location of the event. For instance, using S1 and S2 as reference locations, the murmur location could be of diagnostic value. A third possible use of multiple sensors is to use several sources of the signal when recreating the state space. This would probably give better resistance to measurement noise and, above all, a better embedding of the signal. The major drawback with multiple sensors is that the stethoscope would not be as convenient to use anymore. Further, if additional sensors are to be used, conceptually different techniques such as ECG and Doppler ultrasound should be used as well.

8.3.4   Information fusion

Murmurs caused by MI may be confused with murmurs from tricuspid regurgitation. However, by keeping track of the respiratory cycle, these two murmurs can be distinguished from each other since the tricuspid murmur is augmented during inspiration. This is but one example where additional information aids the physician in the diagnosis. Similarly, the respiratory information can come in handy to evaluate the splitting of S2. If the splitting does not vary with inspiration, it is usually because of an atrial septal defect or ventricular septal defect is present [226]. Obviously, the estimated respiration monitor that was investigated in chapter 7 could be of great use when assessing heart diseases as well.

There are many sources of information that may facilitate the decision making in an intelligent stethoscope. A well of usable knowledge can be found in the patient's medical history. Since the recorded PCG signals will probably be stored in an electronic health record in the future, there are no technical obstacles why information should not flow in the other direction as well. Such ideas have already been investigated by Javed et al. [113], however, the ethical considerations in such approaches have yet to be carefully studied.

8.3.5   Model-based signal analysis

If a model can be incorporated in the analysis of the PCG, it is likely that more effective processing schemes can be constructed. For simulation purposes, models such as the ones for S1 and S2 in section 2.6 can be used. There are, however, no models that are flexible and robust enough to describe the entire PCG signal. Model-based signal processing may however be used on more restricted subproblems. One example is the determination of the S2-split. By fitting a model of S2 to the recorded signal, the splitting between the aortic and pulmonary components can be obtained directly from the model parameters. Equation 8.1 provides a rather simple

191

model of S2 consisting of two windowed sinusoids. The sinusoids are defined by their amplitudes A, frequencies ω and phases φ, while the window is implemented as a Gaussian function where m and σ control the location and width of the window, respectively.

$$S_2(t) = A_a sin(\omega_a t + \varphi_a) \cdot \frac{1}{\sigma_a \sqrt{2\pi}} e^{-\frac{(t-m_a)^2}{2\sigma_a^2}} + A_p sin(\omega_p t + \varphi_p) \cdot \frac{1}{\sigma_p \sqrt{2\pi}} e^{-\frac{(t-m_p)^2}{2\sigma_p^2}} \quad (8.1)$$

An efficient method to fit the model to the recorded sound is to minimize the squared error. This can be achieved using a 10-dimensional nonlinear gradient descent algorithm to determine the ten model parameters. An example showing the possibilities of this technique is illustrated in figure 8.3. Also illustrated in the figure is the joint time-frequency representation of S2, where it is possible to measure the split manually. Once the model has been adjusted to fit the recorded signal, the split can be obtained as the difference $m_p - m_a$.

A more futuristic use of cardiovascular models is to emulate different physical phenomena with the aim to gain knowledge about the underlying processes. Advanced biomechanical dynamical models of the heart have been developed [157]. The main flow characteristics of the vortices and eddies predicted by the model can also be verified by in vivo visualizations obtained from MRI [242]. Recent advances in MRI even make it possible to investigate turbulence in vivo by measuring the standard deviation of the blood flow velocity distribution within voxels [55,56]. Using knowledge and data from these kinds of measurements, it might be possible to incorporate more reliable information into models of the heart. In the end, the models might be accurate enough to reproduce the cardiovascular system in such detail that also the accompanying sound field can be modeled. Integration between signal processing and such a model would be capable of directly attributing pathophysiological meaning to the parameters obtained from the signal processing algorithms. Until this model becomes available, state space reconstruction from the PCG signal offers a means of describing the underlying dynamical system in terms of structure and behavior. Throughout this book, the embedding dimension has been determined with Cao's method [38]. Interestingly, obtained d-values have always been fairly constant regardless of the patients' disease state. This implies that the number of differential equations involved in a system model does not change with health status, and that only model parameters differ.

8.3.6   Obstacles

This book contains a number of examples and results showing the potential use of computerized phonocardiography. In the literature, methodologies able to distinguish a large number of different murmurs from each other have been developed and excellent classification results have been presented. If this is the case, why are there no successful commercial products available? There are a number of possible reasons:

1. Many journal articles and conference proceedings are based on PCG data obtained from teaching tapes and data bases used for teaching auscultation.

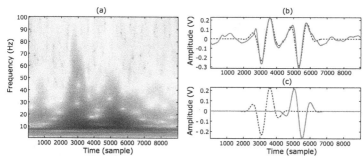

Fig. 8.3: Time-frequency representation of S2 (a). A model of S2 (blue) and the recorded sound signal (red) is given in (b) and the two model components representing A2 and P2 are shown in (c).

The problem is that such data sets contain textbook cases where the signals are nearly noise-free and very typical for the disease at hand. When training a classifier on such signals, it is not very surprising that system performance decreases when real data are used.

2. Many algorithms are designed to separate something pathological from something physiological. In real life, there is always a gray zone that is seldom investigated in published work.

3. Patients (and probably physicians as well) in developed countries do not trust the results of a gadget which is based on something as basic as heart sounds. If a physician tells you that you have a heart murmur, would you settle with anything less than a full echocardiographic investigation?

4. Still no one knows the true origin of the heart sounds. There are two working hypotheses, and the truth is probably somewhere in between. Maybe very accurate cardiac models will bring clarity into this issue.

5. Measurement noise is still a big problem. In a clinical environment the recordings will contain friction rubs, rumbling sounds from the stomach, breathing sounds from the lungs, background noise from the clinic, etc. All of these noise sources influence the recorded sound in a negative way, but a perhaps bigger problem is handling the stethoscope. This is especially a problem with very skinny patients where it can be difficult to get a good contact surface between the ribs. This is a huge setback since the whole idea behind an intelligent stethoscope is that it should be easy to use (perhaps even by the patients in their homes). Firm application of the sensor cannot be stressed enough to achieve high quality recordings.

6. Most studies use independent data sets for training and testing. However, in some cases, the "independent" data were created using the same patients twice. Acquiring two recordings from the same patient does not make these two recordings independent enough so that one recording can be used for training and the other for testing. Such cross validation will obviously give too optimistic results.

8.4   Starting all over again

The first step in many system identification tasks is to assume a black box and carry on with an estimation of this box based on available data. Most of the work in this book as well as in the PCG signal analysis literature has all been based on this concept. Having exploited information about signal morphology, frequency properties, joint time-frequency properties and now even nonlinear signal properties, I am not sure that further research along this line of thought can be brought much further. Instead, I believe that the black box thinking has to be complemented or replaced by a strategy built on a realistic model of the heart. If I was to start all over again, I would have begun with taking massive courses in computational fluid dynamics and dynamical modeling of heart dynamics. Based on a proper model, the sound signal can hopefully be reverse engineered and the full potential of the PCG signal might finally be revealed.

Bibliography

[1] H. D. I. Abarbanel. *Analysis of observed chaotic data.* Springer-Vlg, New York, 1996.

[2] A. E. Abbas. Entropy. In M. Akay, editor, *Wiley Encyclopedia of Biomedical Engineering*, pages 1465–1475. Wiley-Interscience, Wiley and Sons, Hoboken, N.J., 2006.

[3] S. A. Abdallah and N. H. Hwang. Arterial stenosis murmurs: an analysis of flow and pressure fields. *J Acoust Soc Am*, 83(1):318–34, 1988.

[4] P. S. Addison. *Fractals and Chaos: An Illustrated Course.* Taylor & Francis, Gloucester, UK, 1997.

[5] C. Ahlstrom. *Processing of the Phonocardiographic Signal – Methods for the Intelligent Stethoscope.* Licentiate thesis, Linköping, Sweden, May 2006.

[6] C. Ahlstrom. *Nonlinear Phonocardiographic Signal Processing.* PhD thesis, Linköping, Sweden, April 2008.

[7] C. Ahlstrom, K. Höglund, P. Hult, J. Häggström, C. Kvart, and P. Ask. Distinguishing innocent murmurs from murmurs caused by aortic stenosis by recurrence quantification analysis. In *3rd International Conference on Biosignal Processing (ICBP 2006)*, pages 213–218, 2006.

[8] C. Ahlstrom, K. Höglund, P. Hult, J. Häggström, C. Kvart, and P. Ask. Assessing aortic stenosis using sample entropy of the phonocardiographic signal in dogs. *IEEE Transactions on Biomedical Engineering*, 55(8):2107–2109, 2008.

[9] C. Ahlstrom, P. Hult, and P. Ask. Wheeze analysis and detection with nonlinear phase space embedding. In *13th Nordic Baltic Conference, Biomedical Engineering and Medical Physics (NBC05)*, pages 305–306, 2005.

[10] C. Ahlstrom, P. Hult, and P. Ask. Detection of the 3rd heart sound using recurrence time statistics. In *31st International Conference on Acoustics, Speech, and Signal Processing (ICASSP2006)*, pages II:1040–1043, 2006.

[11] C. Ahlstrom, P. Hult, P. Rask, J-E Karlsson, E. Nylander, U. Dahlström, and P. Ask. Feature extraction for systolic heart murmur classification. *Ann Biomed Eng*, 34(11):1666–1677, 2006.

[12] C. Ahlstrom, A. Johansson, P. Hult, and P. Ask. Chaotic dynamics of respiratory sounds. *Chaos, Solitons and Fractals*, 29:1054–1062, 2006.

[13] C. Ahlstrom, A. Johansson, T. Länne, and P. Ask. Noninvasive investigation of blood pressure changes using the pulse wave transit time: a novel approach in the monitoring of hemodialysis patients. *J Artif Organs*, 8:192–197, 2005.

[14] C. Ahlstrom, O. Liljefeldt, P. Hult, and P. Ask. Heart sound cancellation from lung sound recordings using recurrence time statistics and nonlinear prediction. *IEEE Signal Proc Lett*, 12:812–815, 2005.

[15] C. Ahlstrom, T. Länne, P. Ask, and A. Johansson. A method for accurate localization of the first heart sound and possible applications. *Physiol Meas*, 29:417–428, 2008.

[16] M. Akay, Y. M. Akay, W. Welkowitz, and S. Lewkowicz. Investigating the effects of vasodilator drugs on the turbulent sound caused by femoral artery stenosis using short-term fourier and wavelet transform methods. *IEEE Trans Biomed Eng*, 41(10):921–928, 1994.

[17] R. A. Allen, J. A. Schneider, D. M. Davidson, M. A. Winchester, and C. B. Taylor. The covariation of blood pressure and pulse transit time in hypertensive patients. *Psychophysiology*, 18:301–306, 1981.

[18] J. A. Anderson. *An introduction to neural networks*. MIT Press, Cambridge, Massachusetts, 1997.

[19] P. Ask, B. Hok, D. Loyd, and H. Terio. Bio-acoustic signals from stenotic tube flow: state of the art and perspectives for future methodological development. *Med Biol Eng Comput*, 33(5):669–75, 1995.

[20] P. Bao and L. Zhang. Noise reduction for magnetic resonance images via adaptive multiscale products thresholding. *IEEE Trans Med Imag*, 22(9):1089–1099, 2003.

[21] E. Baracca, D. Scorzoni, M. C. Brunazzi, P. Sgobino, L. Longhini, D. Fratti, and C. Longhini. Genesis and acoustic quality of the physiological fourth heart sound. *Acta Cardiol*, 50:23–28, 1995.

[22] A. Bartels and D. Harder. Non-invasive determination of systolic blood pressure by heart sound pattern analysis. *Clin Phys Physiol Meas*, 13:249–256, 1992.

[23] C. Basso, P. R. Fox, K. M. Meurs, J. A. Towbin, A. W. Spier, F. Calabrese, B. J. Maron, and G. Thiene. Arrhythmogenic right ventricular cardiomyopathy causing sudden cardiac death in boxer dogs. *Circulation*, 109:1180–1185, 2004.

[24] K. Bendjelid, P. M. Suter, and J. A. Romand. The respiratory change in pre-ejection period: a new method to predict fluid responsiveness. *J Appl Physiol*, 96:337–342, 2004.

[25] R. M. Berne and M. N. Levy. *Cardiovascular Physiology*. Mosby, St. Louise, Missouri, 7. edition, 1997.

[26] M. Bier, O. W. Day, and D. W. Pravica. Murmurs and noise caused by arterial narrowing - theory and clinical practice. *Fluctuation and Noise Letters*, 6(4):L415–L425, 2006.

[27] M. Bland. *An introduction to medical statistics*. Oxford University Press, Oxford, GB, 3. edition, 2000.

[28] J. A. Bloom. *Monitoring of respiration and circulation*. CRC Press, Boca Raton, Florida, 2004.

[29] R. O. Bonow and E. Braunwald. Valvular heart disease. In D. P. Zipes and E. E. Braunwald, editors, *Braunwald's heart disease: a textbook of cardiovascular medicine*, pages 1553–1632. Saunders, Philadelphia.

[30] R. O. et al. Bonow. Acc/aha 2006 guidelines for management of patients with valvular heart disease: executive summary. *Circ*, 114:e84–e231, 2006.

[31] G. J. Borden, K. S. Harris, and L. J. Raphael. *Speech science primer : physiology, acoustics, and perception of speech*. Williams & Wilkins, Baltimore, 3. edition, 1994.

[32] M. Borgarelli, P. Savarino, S. Crosara, R. A. Santilli, D. Chiavegato, M. Poggi, C. Bellino, G. La Rosa, R. Zanatta, J. Haggstrom, and A. Tarducci. Survival characteristics and prognostic variables of dogs with mitral regurgitation attributable to myxomatous valve disease. *J Vet Intern Med*, 22:120–128, 2008.

[33] S. Borokova, R. Burton, and H. Dehling. Consistency of the takens estimator for the correlation dimension. *Ann Appl Prob*, 9:376–390, 1999.

[34] S. Boudaoud, H. Rix, and O. Meste. Integral shape averaging and structural average estimation: a comparative study. *IEEE Trans Sig Proc*, 53:3644–3650, 2005.

[35] R. N. Bracewell. *The Fourier transform and its applications*. McGraw Hill, Boston, 3. edition, 2000.

[36] J. C. Bramwell and A. V. Hill. The velocity of the pulse wave in man. *Proceedings of the Royal Society of London. Series B, Containing Papers of a Biological Character*, 93:298–306, 1922.

[37] D. S. Broomhead, R. Jones, and G. P. King. Topological dimension and local coordinates from time series data. *Phys A*, 20:563–569, 1987.

[38] L. Cao. Practical method for determining the minimum embedding dimension of a scalar time series. *Phys D*, 110:43–50, 1997.

[39] I. Cathers. Neural network assisted cardiac auscultation. *Artif Intell Med*, 7(1):53–66, 1995.

[40] S. Charleston and M. R. Azimi-Sadjadi. Reduced order kalman filtering for the enhancement of respiratory sounds. *IEEE Trans Biomed Eng*, 43(4):421–4, 1996.

[41] S. Charleston, M. R. Azimi-Sadjadi, and R. Gonzalez-Camarena. Interference cancellation in respiratory sounds via a multiresolution joint time-delay and signal-estimation scheme. *IEEE Trans Biomed Eng*, 44(10):1006–19, 1997.

[42] D. Chen, L-G. Durand, and H.C. Lee. Time-frequency analysis of the first heart sound. part 1: Simulation and analysis. *Med Biol Eng Comput*, 35:306–310, 1997.

[43] W. Chen, T. Kobayashi, S. Ichikawa, Y. Takeuchi, and T. Togawa. Continuous estimation of systolic blood pressure using the pulse arrival time and intermittent calibration. *Med Biol Eng Comput*, 38(5):569–574, 2000.

[44] E. Conte, A. Vena, A. Federici, R. Giuliani, and J. P. Zbilut. A brief note on possible detection of physiological singularities in respiratory dynamics by recurrence quantification analysis of lung sounds. *Chaos Solitons Fractals*, 21:869–877, 2004.

[45] C. C. Cornell, M. D. Kittleson, P. Della Torre, J. Häggström, C. W. Lombard, H. D. Pedersen, A. Vollmar, and A. Wey. Allometric scaling of m-mode cardiac measurements in normal adult dogs. *J Vet Intern Med*, 18(3):311–321, 2004.

[46] J. P. de Vos and M. M. Blanckenberg. Automated pediatric cardiac auscultation. *IEEE Trans Biomed Eng*, 54(2):244–52, 2007.

[47] C. G. DeGroff, S. Bhatikar, J. Hertzberg, R. Shandas, L. Valdes-Cruz, and R. L. Mahajan. Artificial neural network-based method of screening heart murmurs in children. *Circulation*, 103(22):2711–2716, 2001.

[48] D. K. Dey, V. Sundh, and B. Steen. Do systolic murmurs predict mortality in the elderly? a 15-year longitudinal population study of 70-year-olds. *Arch Gerontol Geriatr*, 38:191–200, 2004.

[49] R. L. Donnerstein. Continuous spectral analysis of heart murmurs for evaluating stenotic cardiac lesions. *Am J Cardiol*, 64:625–630, 1989.

[50] D. L. Donoho and I. M. Johnstone. Ideal spatial adaptation by wavelet shrinkage. *Biometrika*, 81:425–455, 1994.

[51] M. J. Drinnan, J. Allen, and A. Murray. Relation between heart rate and pulse transit time during paced respiration. *Physiol Meas*, 22(3):425–32, 2001.

[52] K. Dumont. *Experimental and numerical modeling of heart valve dynamics*. PhD thesis, Gent, Belgium, December 2004.

[53] L-G. Durand, Y. E. Langlois, T. Lanthier, R. Chiarella, P. Coppens, S. Carioto, and S. Bertrand-Bradley. Spectral analysis and acoustic transmission of mitral and aortic valve closure sounds in dogs. part 1 modelling the heart/thorax acoustic system. *Med Biol Eng Comp*, 28:269–277, 1990.

[54] L-G. Durand and P. Pibarot. Digital signal processing of the phonocardiogram: review of the most recent advancements. *CRC Critical Reviews Biomed Eng*, 23:163–219, 1995.

[55] P. Dyverfeldt, J-P. Escobar Kvitting, A. Sigfridsson, J. Engvall, A. F. Bolger, and T. Ebbers. Assessment of fluctuating velocities in disturbed cardiovascular blood flow: In-vivo feasibility of generalized phase-contrast MRI. *Accepted for publication in Magn Reson Med*, 2008.

[56] P. Dyverfeldt, A. Sigfridsson, J-P. Kvitting, and T. Ebbers. Quantification of intravoxel velocity standard deviation and turbulence intensity by generalizing phase-contrast MRI. *Magn Reson Med*, 56:850–858, 2006.

[57] J-P. Eckmann, S. O. Kamphorst, and D. Ruelle. Recurrence plots of dynamical systems. *Europhys. Lett.*, 4:973–977, 1987.

[58] J-P. Eckmann and D. Ruelle. Ergodic theory of chaos and strange attractors. *Rev Mod Phys*, 57:617–656, 1985.

[59] J-P. Eckmann and D. Ruelle. Fundamental limitations for estimating dimensions and lyapunov exponents in dynamical systems. *Phys D*, 56:185–187, 1992.

[60] A. Egenvall, B. N. Bonnett, Å. Hedhammar, and P. Olson. Mortality in over 350,000 insured swedish dogs from 1995-2000: Ii. breed-specific age and survival patterns and relative risk for causes of death. *Avta Vet Scand*, 46:121–136, 2005.

[61] M. El-Segaier. *Digital analysis of cardiac acoustic signals in children*. PhD thesis, Lund, Sweden, April 2007.

[62] M. El-Segaier, O. Lilja, S. Lukkarinen, L. Sornmo, R. Sepponen, and E. Pesonen. Computer-based detection and analysis of heart sound and murmur. *Ann Biomed Eng*, 33:937–942, 2005.

[63] J. B. Elsner and A. A. Tsonis. *Singular Spectrum Analysis: A new tool in time series analysis*. Plenum, New York, 1996.

[64] D. Erdogmus and J. C. Principe. From linear adaptive filtering to nonlinear information processing. *IEEE Signal Processing Magazine*, 23(6):14–33, 2006.

[65] R. Esteller, G. Vachtsevanos, J. Echauz, and B. Litt. A comparison of waveform fractal dimension algorithms. *IEEE Trans Circ Syst*, 48:177–183, 2001.

[66] P. Findlen. A history of the heart.
Internet online, 23 October 2007.
http://www.stanford.edu/class/history13/earlysciencelab/body/heartpages/.

[67] H. Fletcher and W. Munson. Loudness, its definition, measurement and calculation. *J Acoust Soc Am*, 5:82–108, 1933.

[68] D. Flores-Tapia, Z. M. Moussavi, and G. Thomas. Heart sound cancellation based on multiscale products and linear prediction. *IEEE Trans Biomed Eng*, 54(2):234–243, 2007.

[69] D. Franchi, R. Bedini, F. Manfredini, S. Berti, G. Palagi, S. Ghione, and A. Ripoli. Blood pressure evaluation based on arterial pulse wave velocity. *Computers in cardiology*, 23:108–111, 1996.

[70] A. M. Fraser and H. L. Swinney. Independent coordinates for strange attractors from mutual information. *Physical Review A*, 33(2):1134–1140, 1986.

[71] R. Gamboa, P. G. Hugenholtz, and A. S. Nadas. Accuracy of the phonocardiogram in assessing severity of aortic and pulmonic stenosis. *Circulation*, 30:35–46, 1964.

[72] J. B. Gao. Recurrence time statistics for chaotic systems and their applications. *Phys. Rev. Lett.*, 83:3178–3181, 1999.

[73] J. B. Gao, Y. Cao, L. Gu, J. G. Harris, and J. C. Principe. Detection of weak transitions in signal dynamics using recurrence time statistics. *Phys Lett A*, 317:64–72, 2003.

[74] N. A. Gershenfeld and A. W. Weigend. The future of time series. In N. A. Gershenfeld and A. W. Weigend, editors, *Time series prediction: Forecasting the future and understanding the past*, pages 1–70. Westview Press, Boulder, CO.

[75] D. Gill, N. Gavrieli, and N. Intrator. Detection and identification of heart sounds using homomorphic envelogram and self-organizing probabilistic model. In *Computers in Cardiology, 2005*, pages 957–960, 2005.

[76] J. Gnitecki and Z. Moussavi. Variance fractal dimension trajectory as a tool for hear sound localization in lung sounds recordings. In *Engineering in Medicine and Biology Society, 2003. Proceedings of the 25th Annual International Conference of the IEEE*, volume 3, pages 2420–2443, 2003.

[77] J. Gnitecki and Z. M. Moussavi. Separating heart sounds from lung sounds. accurate diagnosis of respiratory disease depends on understanding noises. *IEEE Eng Med Biol Mag*, 26(1):20–29, 2007.

[78] J. Gnitecki, Z. M. Moussavi, and H. Pasterkamp. Diagnostic potential in state space parameters of lung sounds. *Med Biol Eng Comp*, 46(1):93–99, 2007.

[79] A. L. Goldberger. Fractal mechanisms in the electrophysiology of the heart. *IEEE Eng Med Biol Mag*, 26:47–52, 1992.

[80] P. Gonçalves, P. Flandrin, and E. Chassande-Mottin. Time-frequency methods in time-series data analysis. In *Second Workshop on Gravitational Wave Data Analysis*, pages 35–46, 1997.

[81] L. Gould, S. J. Ettinger, and A. F. Lyon. Intensity of the first heart sound and arterial pulse in mitral insufficiency. *Dis Chest*, 53:545–549, 1968.

[82] R. B. Govindan, J. D. Wilson, H. Eswaran, C. L. Lowery, and H. Preißl. Revisiting sample entropy analysis. *Phys A*, 376:158–164, 2007.

[83] G. Granlund and H. Knutsson. *Signal processing for computer vision.* Kluwer, Dordrecht, 1995.

[84] P. Grassberger and I. Procaccia. Estimation of the kolmogorov entropy from a chaotic signal. *Phys Rev A*, 28:2591–2593, 1983.

[85] M. C. Grenier, K. Gagnon, J. Genest, J. Durand, and L. G. Durand. Clinical comparison of acoustic and electronic stethoscopes and design of a new electronic stethoscope. *Am J Cardiol*, 81(5):653–656, 1998.

[86] C. N. Gupta, R. Palaniappan, S. Swaminathan, and S. M. Krishnan. Neural network classification of homomorphic segmented heart sounds. *Applied Soft Computing*, 7(1):286–297, 2007.

[87] F. Gustafsson. *Adaptive Filtering and Change Detection.* Wiley, England, 2000.

[88] I. Guyon and A. Elisseeff. An introduction to variable and feature selection. *J Mach Learn Res*, 3:1157–1182, 2003.

[89] L. J. Hadjileontiadis. Higher-order statistics. In M. Akay, editor, *Wiley Encyclopedia of Biomedical Engineering*, pages 1871–1886. Wiley-Interscience, Wiley and Sons, Hoboken, N.J., 2006.

[90] L. J. Hadjileontiadis and S. M. Panas. Adaptive reduction of heart sounds from lung sounds using fourth-order statistics. *IEEE Trans Biomed Eng*, 44(7):642–8, 1997.

[91] L. J. Hadjileontiadis and S. M. Panas. Discrimination of heart sounds using higher-order statistics. In *Engineering in Medicine and Biology Society, 1997. EMBS '97. 19th Annual International Conference of the IEEE*, pages 1138–1141, 1997.

[92] A. Haghighi-Mood and J. N. Torry. A sub-band energy tracking algorithm for heart sound segmentation. In *Computers in Cardiology, 1995*, pages 501–504, 1995.

[93] A. Haghighi-Mood and J. N. Torry. Time-varying filtering of the first and second heart sounds. In *Engineering in Medicine and Biology Society, 1996. EMBS '96. 18th Annual International Conference of the IEEE*, pages 950–951, 1996.

[94] M. Han, Y Liu, J Xi, and W. Guo. Noise smoothing for nonlinear time series using wavelet soft threshold. *IEEE Sig Proc Lett*, 14:62–65, 2007.

[95] F. Hasfjord. Heart sound analysis with time dependent fractal dimensions. Master's thesis, Linköping, Sweden, February 2004.

[96] H. Hassanpour, M. Mesbah, and B. Boashash. Time-frequency feature extraction of newborn EEG seizure using svd-based techniques. *Eurasip J Appl Sig Proc*, 16:2544–2554, 2004.

[97] J. Hawkins. *On intelligence*. Times Books, New York, 2004.

[98] R. Heiene, A. Indrebø, C. Kvart, H. M. Skaalnes, and A. K. Ulstad. Prevalence of murmurs consistent with aortic stenosis among boxer dogs in norway and sweden. *The Vet Rec*, 5:152–156, 2000.

[99] J. Häggström, C. Kvart, and K. Hansson. Heart sounds and murmurs: changes related to the severity of chronic valvular disease in the cavalier king charles spaniel. *J Vet Int Med*, 9(2):75–85, 1995.

[100] J. Häggström, C. Kvart, and H. D. Pedersen. Acquired valvular heart disease. In S.J. Ettinger and E. C. Felman, editors, *Textbook of veterinary internal medicine*, pages 1022–1039. Elsevier Saunders, St. Louis, Missouri, 2005.

[101] K. Höglund, C. Ahlstrom, J. Häggström, P. Ask, P. Hult, and C. Kvart. Time-frequency and complexity analysis – a new method for differentiation of innocent murmurs from heart murmurs caused by aortic stenosis in boxer dogs. *A J Vet Res*, 68:962–969, 2007.

[102] M. J. Hinich. Testing for gaussianity and linearity of a stationary time series. *J Time Series Analysis*, 3:169–176, 1982.

[103] J. Hisdal, K. Toska, T. Flatebo, B. Waaler, and L. Walloe. Regulation of arterial blood pressure in humans during isometric muscle contraction and lower body negative pressure. *Eur J Appl Physiol*, 91:336–341, 2004.

[104] F. Hlawatsch and G. F. Boudreaux-Bartels. Linear and quadratic time-frequency signal representations. *IEEE Signal Processing Magazine*, 9(2):21–68, 1992.

[105] D. Hoyer, B. Pompe, K. H. Chon, H. Hardraht, C. Wisher, and U. Zweiner. Mutual information function assesses autonomic information flow of heart rate dynamics at different time scales. *IEEE Trans Biomed Eng*, 52:584–592, 2005.

[106] N. E. Huang, Z. Shen, S. R. Long, M. C. Wu, H. H. Shih, Q. Zheng, N.-C. Yen, C. C. Tung, and H. H. Liu. The empirical mode decomposition and the hilbert spectrum for nonlinear and non-stationary time series analysis. *Royal Soc London Proc Series A*, 454:903–995, 1996.

[107] P. Hult. *Bioacoustic principles used in monitoring and diagnostic applications*. PhD thesis, Linköping, Sweden, November 2002.

[108] P. Hult, T. Fjällbrant, K. Hilden, U. Dahlström, B. Wranne, and P. Ask. Detection of the third heart sound using a tailored wavelet approach: method verification. *Med Biol Eng Comput*, 43:212–217, 2005.

[109] P. Hult, T. Fjällbrant, B. Wranne, and P. Ask. Detection of the third heart sound using a tailored wavelet approach. *Med Biol Eng Comput*, 42:253–258, 2004.

[110] J. O. Humphries and J. M. Criley. Comparison of heart sounds and murmurs in man and animals. *Annals of the New York Academy of Sciences*, 127:341–353, 1965.

[111] A. Hyvärinen, J. Karhunen, and E. Oja. *Independent component analysis*. Wiley, New York, 2001.

[112] A. Iwata, N. Ishii, N. Suzumura, and K. Ikegaya. Algorithm for detecting the first and the second heart sounds by spectral tracking. *Med Biol Eng Comput*, 18(1):19–26, 1980.

[113] F. Javed, P. A. Venkatachalam, and A. F. Hani. Knowledge based system with embedded intelligent heart sound analyser for diagnosing cardiovascular disorders. *J Med Eng Technol*, 31(5):341–350, 2007.

[114] Z. Jiang, S. Choi, and H. Wang. A new approach on heart murmurs classification with svm technique. In Samjin Choi, editor, *Information Technology Convergence, 2007. ISITC 2007. International Symposium on*, pages 240–244, 2007.

[115] A. Johansson, C. Ahlstrom, T. Lanne, and P. Ask. Pulse wave transit time for monitoring respiration rate. *Med Biol Eng Comput*, 44(6):471–478, 2006.

[116] A. Johansson and B. Hök. Sensors for respiratory monitoring. In P. Å. Öberg, T. Togawa, and F. Spelman, editors, *Sensors in medicine and health care*, pages 161–186. Wiley-VCH, Weinheim.

[117] H. Jung, J. W. Choi, and C. G. Park. Asymmetric flows of non-newtonian fluids in symmetric stenosed artery. *Korea-Australia Rheology Journal*, 16(2):101–108, 2004.

[118] H. Kantz and T. Schreiber. *Nonlinear time series analysis*. Cambridge University Press, Cambridge, UK, 2. edition, 2004.

[119] A. M. Katz. *Physiology of the heart*. Raven Press, New York, 2. edition, 1992.

[120] M. J. Katz. Fractals and the analysis of waveforms. *Comput Biol Med*, 40:517–526, 1988.

[121] S. H. Kellert. *In the wake of chaos*. The Univertity of Chicago Press, Chicago, US, 1993.

[122] R. D. Kienle. Aortic stenosis. In M. D. Kittleson and R. D. Kienle, editors, *Small animal cardiovascular medicine*, pages 260–272. Mosby, St. Louis, MO, 1998.

[123] D. Kim and M. E. Tavel. Assessment of severity of aortic stenosis through time-frequency analysis of murmur. *Chest*, 124:1638–1644, 2003.

[124] W. Kinsner. Batch and real-time computation of a fractal dimension based on variance of a time series. Technical Report DEL94-6, Dept. of Electrical & Computer Eng., University of Manitoba, Winnipeg, Canada, June 1994.

[125] B. U. Kohler, C. Hennig, and R. Orglmeister. The principles of software qrs detection. *IEEE Eng Med Biol Mag*, 21:42–57, 2002.

[126] A. N. Kolmogorov. The local-structure of turbulence in incompressible viscous-fluid for very large reynolds-numbers. *Dokl Akad Nauk SSR*, 30:301–304, 1941.

[127] S. S. Kraman, G. R. Wodicka, G. A. Pressler, and H. Pasterkamp. Comparison of lung sound transducers using a bioacoustic transducer testing system. *J Appl Physiol*, 101:469–476, 2006.

[128] D. Kugiumtzis and N. Christophersen. State space reconstruction: Method of delays vs singular spectrum approach. Technical Report Research report 236, Department of informatics, University of Oslo, Oslo, Norway, February 1997.

[129] C. Kvart and J. Häggsytröm. *Cardiac auscultation and phonocardiography in dogs, horses and cats.* VIN (Veterinary Information Network), Uppsala, Sweden, 2002.

[130] L. D. Landau. On the problem of turbulence. *Doklady Akademii nauk Souiza Sovetskikh Sotsialisticheskikh Respuplik*, 44:339–344, 1944.

[131] P. Lantelme, C. Mestre, M. Lievre, A. Gressard, and H. Milon. Heart rate: an important confounder of pulse wave velocity assessment. *Hypertension*, 39(6):1083–1087, 2002.

[132] A. Leatham. *Auscultation of the Heart and Phonocardiography.* Churchill Livingstone, New York, 1975.

[133] L. B. Lehmkuhl, J. D. Bonagura, D. E. Jones, and R. L. Stepien. Comparison of catheterization and doppler-derived pressure gradients in a canine model of subaortic stenosis. *J Am Soc Echocardiogr*, 8:611–620, 1995.

[134] R. J. Lehner and R. M. Rangayyan. A three-channel microcomputer system for segmentation and characterization of the phonocardiogram. *IEEE Trans Biomed Eng*, 34(6):485–489, 1987.

[135] T. S. Leung, P. R. White, W. B. Collis, E. Brown, and A. P. Salmon. Analysing paediatric heart murmurs with discriminant analysis. In *Engineering in Medicine and Biology society, 1998. Proceedings of the 20th Annual International Conference of the IEEE*, volume 3, pages 1628–1631, 1998.

[136] T. S. Leung, P. R. White, W. B. Collis, E. A. Brown E. Brown, and A. P. A. Salmon A. P. Salmon. Characterisation of paediatric heart murmurs using self-organising map. In P. R. White, editor, *Engineering in Medicine and*

Biology Society, 1999. EMBS '99. 21st Annual International Conference of the IEEE, volume 2, page 926, 1999.

[137] H. Liang, H. Liang, and I. Hartimo. A heart sound feature extraction algorithm based on wavelet decomposition and reconstruction. In I. Hartimo, editor, *Engineering in Medicine and Biology Society, 1998. EMBS '97. 20th Annual International Conference of the IEEE*, volume 3, pages 1539–1542, 1998.

[138] H. Liang, S. Lukkarinen, and I. Hartimo. Heart sound segmentation algorithm based on heart sound envelogram. In *Computers in Cardiology 1997*, pages 105–108, 1997.

[139] H. Liang, L. Sakari, and H. Iiro. A heart sound segmentation algorithm using wavelet decomposition and reconstruction. In *Engineering in Medicine and Biology society, 1997. Proceedings of the 19th Annual International Conference of the IEEE*, volume 4, pages 1630–1633, 1997.

[140] L. Ljung. *System identification: theory for the user*. Prentice Hall, Upper Saddle River, N.J., 2. edition, 1999.

[141] I. Ljungvall, C. Ahlstrom, K. Höglund, P. Hult, C. Kvart, M. Borgarelli, P. Ask, and J. Häggström. Assessing mitral regurgitation attributable to myxomatous mitral valve disease in dogs using signal analysis of heart sounds and murmurs. *Accepted for publication in A J Vet Res*, 2008.

[142] T. Ölmez and Z. Dokur. Classification of heart sounds using an artificial neural network. *Pattern Recogn Lett*, 24:617–629, 2003.

[143] C. Longhini, E. Barocca, C. Brunazzi, M. Vaccari, L. Longhini, and F. Barbaresi. A new noninvasive method for estimation of pulmonary arterial pressure in mitral stenosis. *Am J Cardiol*, 68:398–401, 1991.

[144] C. Longhini, E. Barocca, D. Mele, C. Fersini, and A. E. Aubert. A mass-spring model hypothesis of the genesis of the physiological third heart sound. *Jpn Heart J*, 30:265–273, 1989.

[145] R. Loudon and R. L. Murphy. Lung sounds. *Am Rev Respir Dis*, 130:663–673, 1984.

[146] P. C. Lu, C. N. Hui, and N. H. Hwang. A model investigation of the velocity and pressure spectra in vascular murmurs. *J Biomech*, 16(11):923–31, 1983.

[147] S. Mallat and W. L. Hwang. Singularity detection and processing with wavelets. *IEEE Trans Inf Theory*, 38(2):617–643, 1992.

[148] D. P. Mandic, M. Chen, T. Gautama, M. M. Van Hulle, and A. Constantinides. On the characterization of the deterministic/stochastic and linear/nonlinear nature of time series. *Royal Soc London Proc Series A*, 464(2093):1141–1160, 2008.

[149] P. Maragos. Fractal dimensions of speech sounds: computation and application to automatic speech recognition. *J Acoust Soc Am*, 105:1925–1932, 1999.

[150] G. V. Marie, C. R. Lo, J. Van Jones, and D. W. Johnston. The relationship between arterial blood pressure and pulse transit time during dynamic and static exercise. *Psychophysiology*, 21(5):521–527, 1984.

[151] M. N. Marinovic and G. Eichmann. Feature extraction and pattern classification in space-spatial frequency domain. In *SPIE Intelligent Robots and Computer Vision*, pages 19–25, 1985.

[152] C. E. Martin, J. A. Shaver, M. E. Thompson, P. S. Reddy, and J. J. Leonard. Direct Correlation of External Systolic Time Intervals with Internal Indices of Left Ventricular Function in Man. *Circulation*, 44(3):419–431, 1971.

[153] J. M. Martinerie, A. M. Albano, A. I. Mees, and P. E. Rapp. Mutual information, strange attractors, and the optimal estimation of dimension. *Phys Rev A*, 45(10):7058–7064, 1992.

[154] N. Marwan, N. Wessel, U. Meyerfeldt, A. Schirdewan, and J. Kurths. Recurrence-plot-based measures of complexity and their application to heart-rate-variability data. *Phys Rev E*, 66:1–8, 2002.

[155] V. A. McKusick, S. A. Talbot, and G. N. Webb. Spectral phonocardiography: problems and prospects in the application of the Bell sound spectrograph to phonocardiography. *Bull john Hopkins Hosp*, 94:187–198, 1954.

[156] J. McNames. A nearest trajectory strategy for time series prediction. In *Int. Workshop on Advanced Black-Box Techniques for Nonlinear Modeling, 1998*, pages 112–128.

[157] D. McQueen and C. Peskin. Heart simulation by an immersed boundary method with formal second-order accuracy and reduced numerical viscosity. In H. Aref and J. W. Philips, editors, *Mechanics for a New Mellennium*, pages 429–444. Springer, Netherlands, 2000.

[158] N. J. Mehta and I. A. Khan. Third heart sound: genesis and clinical importance. *Int J Cardiol*, 97(2):183–186, 2004.

[159] A. Miller, R. S. Lees, J. P. Kistler, and W. M. Abbott. Spectral analysis of arterial bruits (phonoangiography): experimental validation. *Circulation*, 61(3):515–520, 1980.

[160] S. Minfen and S. Lisha. The analysis and classification of phonocardiogram based on higher-order spectra. In *Proc. of the IEEE-SP, Higher-Order Statistics 1997*, pages 29–33.

[161] E. Moreyra, B. L. Segal, and H. Shimada. The murmurs of mitral regurgitation. *Chest*, 55(1):49–53, 1969.

[162] T. Mori, N. Ohnishi, K. Sekioka, T. Nakano, and H. Takezawa. Power spectrum of heart murmurs: special reference to mitral regurgitant murmurs. *J Cardiogr*, 16(4):977–986, 1986.

[163] Z. Moussavi. *Fundamentals of respiratory sounds and analysis*. Morgan & Claypool, San Rafael, Californa, 1. edition, 2007.

[164] J. A. Máttar, W. C. Shoemaker, D. Diament, A. Lomar, A. C. Lopes, E. De Freitas, F. P. Stella, and L. A. Factore. Systolic and diastolic time intervals in the critically ill patient. *Crit Care Med*, 19:1382–1386, 1991.

[165] D. B. Newlin. Relationships of pulse transmission times to pre-ejection period and blood pressure. *Psychophysiology*, 18(3):316–321, 1981.

[166] V. Nigam and R. Priemer. Accessing heart dynamics to estimate durations of heart sounds. *Physiol Meas*, 26(6):1005–18, 2005.

[167] C. L. Nikias and J. M. Mendel. Signal processing with higher-order spectra. *IEEE Signal Processing Magazine*, 10(6):10–37, 1993.

[168] M. Nitzan, B. Khanokh, and Y. Slovik. The difference in pulse transit time to the toe and finger measured by photoplethysmography. *Physiol Meas*, 23(1):85–93, 2002.

[169] R. B. Northrop. *Noninvasive instrumentation and measurement in medical diagnosis*. CRC Chapman & Hall, England, 2002.

[170] H. Nygaard, L. Thuesen, J. M. Hasenkam, E. M. Pedersen, and P. K. Paulsen. Assessing the severity of aortic valve stenosis by spectral analysis of cardiac murmurs (spectral vibrocardiography). Part I: Technical aspects. *J Heart Valve Dis*, 2(4):454–467, 1993.

[171] M. S. Obaidat. Phonocardiogram signal analysis: techniques and performance comparison. *J Med Eng Technol*, 17:221–227, 1993.

[172] M. R. O'Grady, D. Ll Holmberg, C. W. Miller, and J. R. Cockshutt. Canine congenital aortic stenosis: A review of the literature and commentary. *Can Vet J*, 30:811–815, 1989.

[173] H. Olsen, E. Vernersson, and T. Länne. Cardiovascular response to acute hypovolemia in relation to age. Implications for orthostasis and hemorrhage. *Am J Physiol Heart Circ Physiol*, 278(1):H222–232, 2000.

[174] R. A. O'Rourke, V. Fuster, R. W. Alexander, R. Roberts, S. B. King, I. Nash, and E. N. Prystowsky. *Hurst's The Heart Manual of Cardiology*. McGraw-Hill Professional, New York, 11. edition, 2005.

[175] C. M. Otto. Valvular aortic stenosis: disease severity and timing of intervention. *J Am Coll Cardiol*, 47:2141–2151, 2006.

[176] H. Packard, N, J.P. Crutchfield, J. D. Farmer, and R. S. Shaw. Geometry from a time series. *Phys Rev Lett*, 45(9):712–716, 1980.

[177] U. Parlitz. Nonlinear time-series analysis. In J. A. K. Suykens and J. Vandewalle, editors, *Nonlinear modeling: advanced black-box techniques*, pages 209–239. Kluwer Academic Publishers, Boston, 1998.

[178] S. A. Pavlopoulos, A. C. Stasis, and E. N. Loukis. A decision tree–based method for the differential diagnosis of aortic stenosis from mitral regurgitation using heart sounds. *Biomed Eng Online*, 3(1):21, 2004.

[179] R. A. Payne, C. N. Symeonides, and S. R. J. Maxwell. Pulse transit time measured from the ECG: an unreliable marker of beat-to-beat blod pressure. *J Appl Physiol*, 100:136–141, 2006.

[180] H. D. Pedersen and J. Häggström. Mitral valve prolapse in the dog: a model of mitral valve prolapse in man. *Cardiovasc Res*, 47:234–243, 2000.

[181] A. N. Pelech. The physiology of cardiac auscultation. *Pediatr Clin North Am*, 51:1515–1535, 2004.

[182] S. M. Pincus. Approximate entropy as a measure of system complexity. *Proc Natl Acad Sci USA*, 88:2297–2301, 1991.

[183] S. M. Pincus and Goldberger. Al L. Physiological time series analysis: what does regularity quantify? *Am J Physiol*, 266:1643–1656, 1994.

[184] D. J. Pitson, N. Chhina, S. Kniijn, M. van Herwaaden, and J. R. Stradling. Mechanism of pulse transit time lengthening during inspiratory effort. *J Ambul Monit*, 8:101–105, 1995.

[185] D. J. Pitson, A. Sandell, R. van den Hout, and J. R. Stradling. Use of pulse transit time as a measure of inspiratory effort in patients with obstructive sleep apnoea. *Eur Respir J*, 8(10):1669–1674, 1995.

[186] D. J. Pitson and J. R. Stradling. Value of beat-to-beat blood pressure changes, detected by pulse transit time, in the management of the obstructive sleep apnoea/hypopnoea syndrome. *Eur Respir J*, 12(3):685–692, 1998.

[187] M. H. Pollak and P. A. Obrist. Aortic-radial pulse transit time and ECG Q-wave to radial pulse wave interval as indices of beat-by-beat blood pressure change. *Psychophysiology*, 20(1):21–28, 1983.

[188] B. Pompe. Measuring statistical dependences in a time-series. *Journal of Statistical Physics*, 73(3-4):587–610, 1993.

[189] M. T. Pourazad, Z. Moussavi, and G. Thomas. Heart sound cancellation from lung sound recordings using time-frequency filtering. *Med Biol Eng Comput*, 44(3):216–25, 2006.

[190] R. J. Povinelli, M. T. Johnson, A. C. Lindgren, F. M. Roberts, and J. Ye. Statistical models of reconstructed phase spaces for signal classification. *IEEE Trans Sig Proc*, 54(6):2178–2186, 2006.

[191] R. J. Povinelli, M. T. Johnson, A. C. Lindgren, and J. Ye. Time series classfication using gaussian mixture models of reconstructed phase spaces. *IEEE Trans Knowl Data Eng*, 16:779–783, 2004.

[192] P. Pudil, J. Novovicova, and J. Kittler. Floating search methods in feature-selection. *Patt Recogn Lett*, 15:1119–1125, 1994.

[193] R. L. Pyle. Interpreting low-intensity cardiac murmurs in dogs predisposed to subaortic stenosis. *J Am Anim Hosp Assoc*, 36:379–382, 2000.

[194] M. A. Quinones, C. M. Otto, M. Stoddard, A. Waggoner, and W. A. Zoghbi. Recommendations for quantification of doppler echocardiography: a report from the doppler quantification task force of the nomenclature and standards committee of the american society of echocardiography. *J Am Soc Echocardiogr*, 15:167–184, 2002.

[195] M. L. V. Quyen, M. Chavez, D. Rudrauf, and J. Martinerie. Exploring the nonlinear dynamics of the brain. *J Physiol*, 97:629–639, 2003.

[196] P. Ramanand, V. P. Nampoori, and R. Sreenivasan. Complexity quantification of dense array EEG using sample entropy analysis. *J Integr Neurosci*, 3:343–358, 2004.

[197] I. A. Rezek and S. J. Roberts. Stochastic complexity measures for physiological signal analysis. *IEEE Trans Biomed Eng*, 45(9):1186 – 1191, 1998.

[198] J. S. Richman and J. R. Moorman. Physiological time-series analysis using approximate entropy and sample entropy. *Am J Phys - Heart and Circ Phys*, 278:H2039–H2049, 2000.

[199] S. Roweis and L. Saul. Nonlinear dimensionality reduction by locally linear embedding. *Science*, 290:2323–2326, 2000.

[200] D Ruelle and F. Takens. On the nature of turbulence. *Communications in Mathematical Physics*, 20:167–192, 1971.

[201] M. Rugolotto, C. P. Chang, B. Hu, I. Schnittger, and D. H. Liang. Clinical use of cardiac ultrasound performed with a hand-carried device in patients admitted for acute cardiac care. *Am J Cardiol*, 90:1040–1042, 2002.

[202] Robert F. Rushmer. *Cardiovascular dynamics*. Saunders, London, 4. edition, 1976.

[203] H. N. Sabah and P. D. Stein. Turbulent blood flow in humans: its primary role in the production of ejection murmurs. *Circ Res*, 38:513–525, 1976.

[204] A. H. Sacks, E. G. Tickner, and I. B. Macdonald. Criteria for the onset of vascular murmurs. *Circ Res*, 29(3):249–256, 1971.

209

[205] H. E. Schepers, J. H. G. M. van Beek, and J. B. Bassingthwaighte. Four methods to estimate the fractal dimension from self-affine signals. *IEEE Trans Biomed Eng*, 11(2):57–64, 1992.

[206] T. Schreiber. Extremely simple nonlinear noise-reduction method. *Phys Rev E*, 47:2401–2404, 1993.

[207] T. Schreiber. Interdisciplinary application of nonlinear time series methods - the generalized dimensions. *Physics reports*, 308:1–64, 1999.

[208] T. Schreiber and A. Schmitz. Surrogate time series. *Physica D*, 142:346–382, 2000.

[209] S. J. Shah and A. D. Michaels. Hemodynamic correlates of the third heart sound and systolic time intervals. *Congest Heart Fail*, 12(4 Suppl 1):8–13, Jul 2006.

[210] Z. Sharif, M. S. Zainal, A. Z. Sha'ameri, and S. H. S. A. Salleh S. H. S. Salleh. Analysis and classification of heart sounds and murmurs based on the instantaneous energy and frequency estimations. In M. S. Zainal, editor, *TENCON 2000*, volume 2, pages 130–134, 2000.

[211] H. Shino, H. Shino, H. Yoshida, K. Yana, K. A. Harada K. Harada, J. A. Sudoh J. Sudoh, and E. A. Harasewa E. Harasewa. Detection and classification of systolic murmur for phonocardiogram screening detection and classification of systolic murmur for phonocardiogram screening. In H. Yoshida, editor, *Engineering in Medicine and Biology Society, 1996. EMBS '96. 18th Annual International Conference of the IEEE*, volume 1, pages 123–124, 1996.

[212] C. Shub. Echocardiography or auscultation? how to evaluate systolic murmurs. *Can Fam Physician*, 49:163–167, 2003.

[213] R. K. Sinha, Y. Aggarwal, and B. N. Das. Backpropagation artificial neural network classifier to detect changes in heart sound due to mitral valve regurgitation. *J Med Syst*, 31(3):205–209, 2007.

[214] D. Smith and E. Craige. Heart sounds: Toward a consensus regarding their origin. *Am J Noninvas Cardiol*, 2:169–179, 1988.

[215] A. R. A. Sovijärvi, L. P. Malmberg, G. Charbonneau, J. Vanderschoot, F. Dalmasso, C. Sacco, M. Rossi, and J. E. Earis. Characteristics of breath sounds and adventitious respiratory sounds. *Eur Respir Rev*, 10:591–596, 2000.

[216] J. C. Sprott. *Chaos and time-series analysis*. Oxford University Press, Oxford, Great Britain, 2003.

[217] L. Sörnmo and P. Laguna. *Bioelectrical signal processing in cardiac and neurological applications*. Elsevier, New York, 2005.

[218] J. Stark. Observing complexity, seeing simplicity. *Royal Soc London Proc Series A*, 358:41–61, 2000.

[219] B. F. Stewart, D. Siscovick, B. K. Lind, J. M. Gardin, J. S. Gottdiener, V. E. Smith, D. W. Kitzman, and C. M. Otto. Clinical factors associated with calcific aortic valve disease. cardiovascular health study. *J Am Coll Cardiol*, 29:630–634, 1997.

[220] R. G. Stockwell, L. Mansinha, and R. P. Lowe. Localization of the complex spectrum: The s transform. *IEEE Tran Sig Proc*, 44:998–1001, 1996.

[221] F. Takens. Detecting strange attractors in turbulence. In D. A. Rand and L. S. Young, editors, *Dynamical Systems and Turbulence*, pages 366–381. Springer, Berlin, 1981.

[222] M. E. Tavel. Classification of systolic murmurs: Still in search of a consensus. *Curriculum in Cardiology*, 134:330–336, 1997.

[223] M. E. Tavel and H. Katz. Usefulness of a new sound spectral averaging technique to distinguish an innocent systolic murmur from that of aortic stenosis. *Am J Cardiol*, 95:902–904, 2005.

[224] J. Theiler and S. Eubank. Don't bleach chaotic data. *Chaos*, 3:771–782, 1993.

[225] S. Theodoridis and K. Koutroumbas. *Pattern Recognition*. Academic Press, Amsterdam, Netherlands, 2. edition, 2003.

[226] Ara G. Tilkian and Mary Boudreau Conover. *Understanding heart sounds and murmurs: with an introduction to lung sounds*. Saunders, Philadelphia, 4. edition, 2001.

[227] R. J. Tobin and I. D. Chang. Wall pressure spectra scaling downstream of stenoses in steady tube flow. *J Biomech*, 9(10):633–640, 1976.

[228] S. Tong, Z. Li, Y. Zhu, and N. V. Thakor. Describing the nonstationarity level of neurological signals based on quantifications of time frequency representation. *IEEE Transactions on Biomedical Engineering*, 54:1780–1785, 2007.

[229] I. Turkoglu, A. Arslan, and E Ilkay. An intelligent system for diagnosis of the heart valve diseases with wavelet packet neural networks. *Comp Biol Med*, 33:319–331, 2003.

[230] B. Ph. van Milligen, C. Hidalgo, and E. Sánches. Nonlinear phenomena and intermittency in plasma turbulence. *Phys Rev Lett*, 74(3):395–400, 1995.

[231] L. Vannuccini, J. E. Earis, P. Helistö, B. M. G. Cheetham, M. Rossi, A. R. A. Sovijärvi, and J. Vanderschoot. Capturing and preprocessing of respiratory sounds. *Eur Respir Rev*, 10:616–620, 2000.

[232] A. Varsavsky and I. Mareels. A complete strategy for patient un-specific detection of epileptic seizures using crude estimations of entropy. In *Engineering in Medicine and Biology Society, 2007. Proceedings of the 29th Annual International Conference of the IEEE*, volume 1, pages 6191–6194, 2007.

[233] A. Vena, E. Conte, G. Perchiazzi, A. Federici, R. Giuliani, and J. P. Zbilut. Detection of physiological singularities in respiratory dynamics analyzed by recurrence quantification analysis of tracheal sounds. *Chaos Solitons Fractals*, 22:869–881, 2004.

[234] H. Vermarien. Phonocardiography. In J. G. Webster, editor, *Encyclopedia of medical devices and instrumentation*, pages 278–290. Wiley-Interscience, Wiley and Sons, Hoboken, N.J., 2006.

[235] A. Voss, A. Mix, and T. Hubner. Diagnosing aortic valve stenosis by parameter extraction of heart sound signals. *Ann Biomed Eng*, 33(9):1167–1174, 2005.

[236] H. H. Wayne. *Noninvasive technics in cardiology : The phonocardiogram, apexcardiogram, and systolic time intervals*. Year book medical publishers, Chicago, 1973.

[237] C. L. Webber and J. P. Zbilut. Dynamical assessment of physiological systems and states using recurrence plot strategies. *J Appl Physiol*, 76:965–973, 1994.

[238] C. L. Webber and J. P. Zbilut. Recurrence quantification analysis of nonlinear dynamical systems. In M. A. Riley and G. C. Van Orden, editors, *Tutorials in Contemporary Nonlinear Methods for the Behavioral Sciences*, pages 26–94. National Science Foundation, 2005.

[239] A. M. Weissler, W. S. Harris, and C. D. Schoenfeld. Systolic time intervals in heart failure in man. *Circulation*, 37(2):149–159, 1968.

[240] B. West. Complexity, scaling and fractals in biological signals. In M. Akay, editor, *Wiley Encyclopedia of Biomedical Engineering*, pages 926–939. Wiley-Interscience, Wiley and Sons, Hoboken, N.J., 2006.

[241] J. Whitmire and S. Sarkar. Validation of acoustic-analogy predictions from sound radiated by turbulence. *Phys Fluids*, 12:381–391, 2000.

[242] L. Wigström, T. Ebbers, A. Fyrenius, M. Karlsson, J. Engvall, B. Wranne, and A. F. Bolger. Particle trace visualization of intracardiac flow using time-resolved 3D phase contrast MRI. *Magn Reson Med*, 41:793–799, 1999.

[243] C. D. Woody. Characterization of an adaptive filter for the analysis of variable latency neuroelectric signals. *Med Biol Eng Comput*, 5(6):539–554, 1967.

[244] Y. Xiang and S. K. Tso. Detection and classification of flaws in concrete structure using bispectra and neural networks. *Ndt & E International*, 35:19–27, 2002.

[245] J. Xu, L-G. Durand, and P. Pibarot. Nonlinear transient chirp signal modeling of the aortic and pulmonary components of the second heart sound. *IEEE Trans Biomed Eng*, 47(7):1328–1335, 2000.

[246] J. Xu, L-G. Durand, and P. Pibarot. Extraction of the aortic and pulmonary components of the second heart sound using a nonlinear transient chirp signal model. *IEEE Trans Biomed Eng*, 48(3):277–283, 2001.

[247] A. Yadollahi and Z. M. Moussavi. A robust method for heart sounds localization using lung sounds entropy. *IEEE Trans Biomed Eng*, 53(3):497–502, 2006.

[248] Y. Yazicioglu, T. J. Royston, T. Spohnholtz, B. Martin, F. Loth, and H. S. Bassiouny. Acoustic radiation from a fluid-filled, subsurface vascular tube with internal turbulent flow due to a constriction. *J Acoust Soc Am*, 118(2):1193–209, 2005.

[249] A. P. Yoganathan, R. Gupta, F. E. Udwadia, W. H. Corcoran, R. Sarma, and R. J. Bing. Use of the fast fourier transform in the frequency analysis of the second heart sound in normal man. *Med Biol Eng Comput*, 14:455–460, 1976.

[250] A. P. Yoganathan, R. Gupta, F. E. Udwadia, J. W. Miller, W. H. Corcoran, R. Sarma, J. L. Johnson, and R. J. Bing. Use of the fast fourier transform in the frequency analysis of the first heart sound in normal man. *Med Biol Eng Comput*, 14:69–73, 1976.

[251] W. Yongchareon and D. F. Young. Initiation of turbulence in models of arterial stenoses. *J Biomech*, 12(3):185–96, 1979.

[252] J. P. Zbilut, N. Thomasson, and C. L. Webber. Recurrence quantification analysis as a tool for nonlinear exploration of nonstationary cardiac signals. *Medical Engineering & Physics*, 24:53–60, 2002.

[253] H. Zeller, J. Reinecke, D. Tomm, and H. Rieger. Analysis of the sound caused by pulsatile flow through arterial stenosis. In Thomas Kenner, editor, *Cardiovascular system dynamics: models and measurements*, page 668. Plenum, New York, 1982.

[254] Y-T. Zhang, G. Chan, X-Y. Zhang, and L. Yip. Heart sounds and stethoscopes. In M. Akay, editor, *Wiley Encyclopedia of Biomedical Engineering*, pages 1824–1834. Wiley-Interscience, Wiley and Sons, Hoboken, N.J., 2006.

[255] W. A. et al. Zoghbi. Recommendations for evaluation of the severity of native valvular regurgitation with two-dimensional and doppler echocardiography. *J Am Soc Echocardiogr*, 16:777–802, 2003.

213

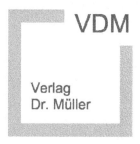

Wissenschaftlicher Buchverlag bietet

kostenfreie

Publikation

von

wissenschaftlichen Arbeiten

Diplomarbeiten, Magisterarbeiten, Master und Bachelor Theses
sowie Dissertationen, Habilitationen und wissenschaftliche Monographien

Sie verfügen über eine wissenschaftliche Abschlußarbeit zu aktuellen oder zeitlosen
Fragestellungen, die hohen inhaltlichen und formalen Ansprüchen genügt,
und haben **Interesse an einer honorarvergüteten Publikation**?

Dann senden Sie bitte erste Informationen über Ihre Arbeit per Email
an info@vdm-verlag.de. Unser Außenlektorat meldet sich umgehend bei Ihnen.

VDM Verlag Dr. Müller Aktiengesellschaft & Co. KG
Dudweiler Landstraße 125a
D - 66123 Saarbrücken

www.vdm-verlag.de

www.ingramcontent.com/pod-product-compliance
Lightning Source LLC
LaVergne TN
LVHW022309060326
832902LV00020B/3351